TAMING JOSH'S DRAGON

A mother's tale of a life too brief.

Debbie Sumner

BALBOA.PRESS
A DIVISION OF HAY HOUSE

Copyright © 2020 Debbie Sumner.

All rights reserved. No part of this book may be used or reproduced by any means, graphic, electronic, or mechanical, including photocopying, recording, taping or by any information storage retrieval system without the written permission of the author except in the case of brief quotations embodied in critical articles and reviews.

Balboa Press books may be ordered through booksellers or by contacting:

Balboa Press
A Division of Hay House
1663 Liberty Drive
Bloomington, IN 47403
www.balboapress.com
1 (877) 407-4847

Because of the dynamic nature of the Internet, any web addresses or links contained in this book may have changed since publication and may no longer be valid. The views expressed in this work are solely those of the author and do not necessarily reflect the views of the publisher, and the publisher hereby disclaims any responsibility for them.

The author of this book does not dispense medical advice or prescribe the use of any technique as a form of treatment for physical, emotional, or medical problems without the advice of a physician, either directly or indirectly. The intent of the author is only to offer information of a general nature to help you in your quest for emotional and spiritual well-being. In the event you use any of the information in this book for yourself, which is your constitutional right, the author and the publisher assume no responsibility for your actions.

Any people depicted in stock imagery provided by Getty Images are models, and such images are being used for illustrative purposes only. Certain stock imagery © Getty Images.

Print information available on the last page.

ISBN: 978-1-9822-4020-2 (sc)
ISBN: 978-1-9822-4019-6 (e)

Balboa Press rev. date: 12/21/2019

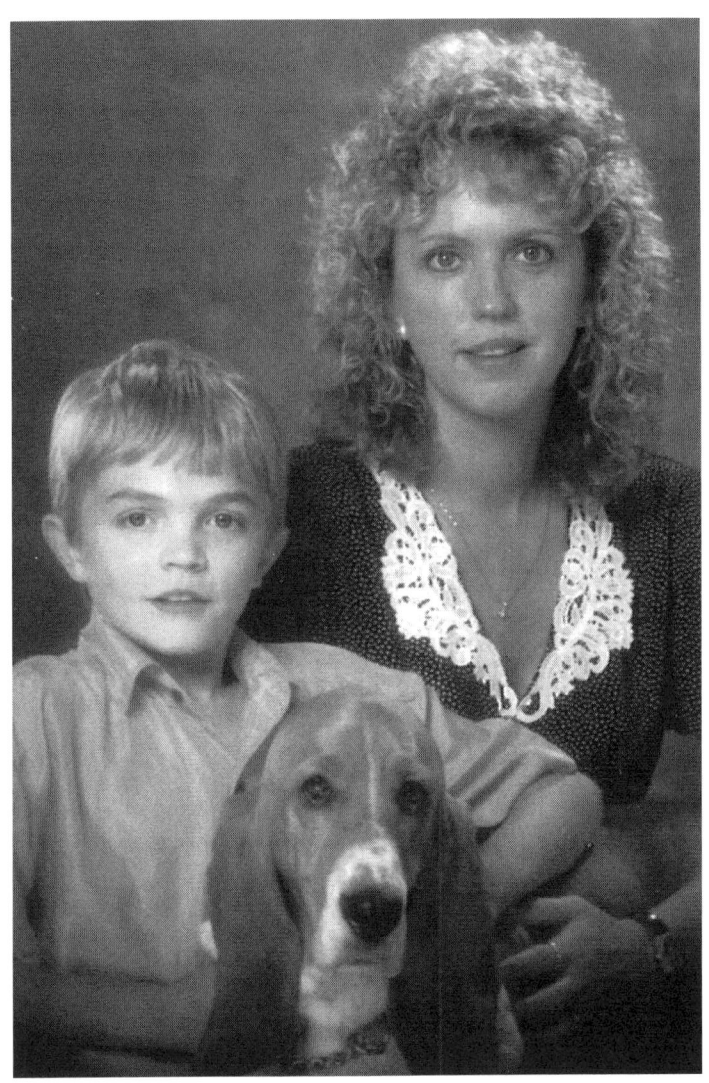

Josh (age 12), Debbie and Cinnamon

THIS DEDICATION IS FOR

- Parents of a child with a life-threatening illness
- Parents of a child who requires or has had a transplant
- Parents who have lost a child
- All the courageous people on the entire spectrum of organ and tissue donation and transplant
  - Organ and tissue donors and their families
  - Patients being considered for transplant
  - Those on the transplant waiting list
  - Organ and tissue transplant recipients
  - Families who lost a loved one following transplant
  - Families who lost a loved one on the waiting list before a donor became available
- And last, but certainly not least, my beloved Josh, angel in my heart and in spirit, without whom my life would have been forever incomplete. Thank you for lessons learned and your teachings of pure love.

Thank you for your interest in my book; God Bless you all; sending you love and hugs from a full heart.

PREFACE

Taming Josh's Dragon is about Josh's life, our transplant experience, our normal day-to-day routines, how together we dealt with his lifelong health challenges, his death and beyond. Yes, there is a "beyond". I consciously made the choice to remain here after lengthy contemplation of and planning for the unthinkable: joining him in the Hereafter.

If you or a loved one faces a lifesaving organ transplant, you may think, "OK, after this is over, my life will return to normal". Well, the truth of the matter is…no, it won't. You must develop your own totally *new* normal. All those years ago we were told, in essence, that you are simply exchanging one health issue for another. A fair trade, indeed, considering that you gain valuable additional time with your loved one.

The many medications must be balanced and monitored through frequent blood work, especially before hospital discharge. There are the biopsies, the checkups, physician appointments and any number of related complications. This information is not meant to discourage the transplant candidate but rather to provide more realistic expectations. Speaking from my own experience, I never liked being blind-sided, so the more knowledgeable I could become prior to transplant, the better prepared and more comfortable I felt it would be. Later I came to question whether this had been a good plan, "being so prepared".

I quickly learned when a loved one is going through the transplant process that it is a whole-family experience. I found myself saying, for example, "When we went for transplant…" and have heard others with the same approach.

My background is in Medical Imaging in the hospital setting. Back when it was simply termed "X-Ray", at age seventeen, I began training at Hamot Hospital School of Radiologic Technology in Erie, Pennsylvania. The terms "Imaging" or "Imaging Services" did not become the preferred designation until much later in my career. Taking my first real job as a radiographer at age nineteen at Warren General Hospital, Warren, Pennsylvania, I gained experience early on in the various modalities of Nuclear Medicine, Ultrasound, CT and Mammography, my specialty being in Radiography. Gradually Imaging Services expanded to include the above-mentioned modalities as well as MRI and various other sub-specialties. I was promoted to a management position at age twenty-nine.

Following a divorce from Josh's father, Jan, in 1993, Josh and I faced the challenge of making it on our own in a new, yet healthier and more peaceful, loving environment. Settling in quickly with Cinnamon, the Basset Hound, we found comfort in each other and in my new-found interest of Country Music that Josh introduced to me. I eventually started to really listen to the lyrics and began to appreciate how many of these songs reflected our life experiences, as well as being chillingly prophetic of those to come. I soon came to love this music genre as much as he did.

My current husband, Ken and I met in 1997 less than two weeks prior to Josh's death. With pride, I remember Ken's surprise when we arrived at my home to find Josh hosing out the garage on his own initiative. Since then, I have tried to relate the wonderful stories we made together so that Ken would have some idea who Josh was. I believe Josh knew at that moment there was going to be someone who would take care of me; he could finally rest easy, the battle surrendered. I truly don't think I would be here today if it hadn't been for Ken's support and understanding during the most difficult time I would ever face.

It is indescribably difficult to lose a child at any age but it even more so when he is young, has fought courageously all his life and it finally seems that the battle has been won. While the years of our journey were quite challenging, they have provided me not only with a better understanding of the power of grief, how it can insidiously work its way deep into your soul and how, in time, it is possible to find your way back into light, laughter, love and life.

This is the story of Josh, a courageous child who struggled his entire life with a chronic, life-threatening lung disease. Following a tough double-lung transplant at the age of 13, it seemed that the road had finally smoothed out for him and he had beaten the ever-present battle for breath itself. Then just four months later came the lung biopsy diagnosis of Obliterative Bronchiolitis (Bronchiolitis Obliterans).[1] Even now, decades after Josh's transplant, that medical term still sends chills through me.

---

[1]. Obliterative bronchiolitis, also known as bronchiolitis obliterans, is a manifestation of chronic allograft rejection, that is, rejection following organ transplantation from another human being. It develops in nearly 50 percent of all patients who receive a lung transplant from an unrelated donor. – My Virtual Medicine Centre

ACKNOWLEDGEMENTS

When beginning this book, I could not appreciate the amount of time that would be required for me to get our story down on paper. It had been fourteen years after his passing when Holly Stimmell said that Josh was communicating to me that I needed to write a book. "A book about what?" I asked. "About us!" was his assured response.

And so it began, thanks to Holly, a cherished local medium. She brought Josh back into my awareness, pushed back the pain and darkness. Holly replaced these with only happiness, delight, laughter and never-ending appreciation for his continued presence in my life. She shed a bright light on the greater meaning of life and did so compassionately, in a delightfully joyful manner. She recognized his inner beauty, humor, strength and the extent to which he shared it with others, in life as well as in spirit. She was the critical element in the writing of this book. Thank you, Holly, for all you are and all you continue to do. I send you love and The White Light of Spirit.

On a more recent visit to Holly, Josh persistently nudged me for completion of this book and insisted that I place my own name in the Acknowledgements section. He was saying, "Mom, I really mean it!" So here it is my dear Josh. Although I don't want to seem boastful in claiming the honor of my motherhood, know that I am humbled and so very proud to have been allowed to share your beautiful and full, yet brief life. I have boundless gratitude for our life's journey and that we decided to travel this meandering and sometime tortuous life path together. Thank you, Josh, for all you have done and the work you continue to do in spirit.

A huge "Thank You" goes out to my kind, compassionate counselor, Frankie Johnson. Eighteen years after Josh's passing, she taught me a very simple method of setting aside the agonizing anxiety and unrelenting heartache surrounding the most difficult portions of this book to discover peace and clear reflection during my creative times. She advised me to simply "Ask Spirit for what you need" and it will be given. Here I also need to acknowledge God for that incredible gift, so easily available only for the asking. Despite this, I still fought to keep it together, especially while incorporating information from medical records from the various sources, so I found myself setting my manuscript aside for months at a time. Recently I have wondered if I am suffering PTSD symptoms activated by the writing of our memoir.

Terry Darling and her son, Oren Darling, in the earliest stages of this book gave me insights and guidance for a time until, writing about our experiences, I hit my first impenetrable wall of pain and emotion, and at that time, needed to put the manuscript away for several years. I thank you both for your assistance, patience and understanding.

A thank you from the bottom of my heart is offered to my beloved cousin, Sandy Downs, a career R.N. who willingly, with love and enthusiasm, without hesitation, agreed to proofread my manuscript, perhaps a rather daunting task for someone who knew and loved Josh. She shed many tears through my memories.

David McConnell, M.D., Josh's lifelong compassionate pediatrician, kindly agreed to also proofread our story, for which I shall be forever grateful. In addition, thank you for your empathy while working all those years with Josh's challenging and, at times, complicated health problems.

A very special synchronicity led me to Emily A. Kunselman, a local artist. I met Emily through Holly Stimmell, who has one of Emily's paintings hung on her office wall. I firmly believe I was led to Emily for a special reason, or perhaps we were led to each other by Josh's spirit for a common goal. Emily is responsible for the stunning design of my book cover. She has done an incredible job incorporating each of my visions and concepts into the cover.

Another synchronicity led me to Martha D. Dexter, a Graphic Artist and now a new and dear friend who properly digitized my photos and aided a technically challenged mom in meeting her publisher's many requirements.

Finally, to my dear husband Ken, thank you for standing by me during the deepest, darkest, most challenging and painful time of my life. You shared your strength and allowed me to grieve in my own way, and grow from the experience. It took an inordinate amount of patience, as I recognize that it was neither easy nor pleasant dealing with me during what

I now acknowledge as my agonizing growth period. I thank you more than I can say for persevering throughout this writing process. With all of my heart and forever, I love you.

Any errors, omissions or limitations in this book are due solely to myself and not those who assisted me.

INTRODUCTION

In preparation for writing this book, and to help establish a timeline for our story, I obtained many of Josh's medical records from Dr. McConnell and Warren General Hospital. Dr. McConnell assisted me in obtaining Josh's records from Children's Hospital of Pittsburgh. Initially I was not aware of how the review of these hundreds of pages would affect me, immediately and traumatically taking me back to those extremely distressing times. Writing this manuscript, there were months at a time when I was compelled to take a break from those agonizing memories.

I have incorporated into my story many of our difficult medical experiences in order for you, the reader, to understand the extent of Josh's health history. The intention is not to overwhelm you with medical descriptions and terms. Rather, it is an account of the life experiences of a little family, a challenge-strewn voyage through a child's life journey and my discovery of the pure and unconditional love of a precious young boy. This story describes Josh's bold passage along our shared voyage as a lovely child with a strong, resilient spirit, who happened to be burdened with a life-long chronic, life-threatening disease.

For Josh, me, and our story, use of the term "dragon" has multiple layers of meaning. A peeling back of those layers reveals that Josh had had an affinity for dragons since he'd started a Shotokan Karate class at the age of three. Dragons are known to play a large part in Japanese culture; I still have his ferocious-looking silver dragon ring and red-eyed dragon pendant. In addition, his school mascot is a fierce Dragon. Lastly and most importantly, I considered Josh's lifelong battle with lung disease a frightful dragon that needed to be tamed.

I know deep in my soul that writing our story was a collaborative effort from this side of life and from beyond, all beautifully colored with our love. Josh guided my hand as each word went down and I healed more with each emerging, although frequently unbearable, paragraph. He infused his spirit's strength into mine to complete our beautiful, entwined life story. I now ask myself if it is really possible that our love has increased because this tale is finally on paper, helping others to more easily navigate the same tortuous path.

What a precious gift sharing Josh's life was for me. I have learned over the years that he had touched many other lives in an incredibly positive manner as well. I will forever be thankful for the time I had with him and will always treasure the precious memories we made together. I am so very grateful to have known him and am honored to have been bestowed the title "mother" of this delightful, courageous child and will hold his beautiful spirit forever in my mind and my heart. Thank you, God, for this precious child-gift, a soul-teacher then, now and forever.

I have only just recently understood that the worst day of my life brought me a depth of appreciation I could never before have imagined. It gave me a perspective from the place of gratitude for being blessed to have known this child, for having been gifted fifteen-and-a-half brief—yet immeasurably valuable—years with him. Most importantly, I am grateful for the significant life-lessons of unending joy, selflessness and incredibly profound love of life that he taught and continues to teach me. Until we are together again, Josh, I love you forever and always.

CONTENTS

Chapter 1	A New Little Person	1
Chapter 2	Watching Josh Improve	7
Chapter 3	A Smile!	15
Chapter 4	Hospital Admissions	21
Chapter 5	Let the Fun Begin!	25
Chapter 6	A Young Josh	31
Chapter 7	The Elementary Years	37
Chapter 8	Continuing Health Issues	41
Chapter 9	A Sad Split	43
Chapter 10	Challenges	47
Chapter 11	Transplant Evaluation	51
Chapter 12	Preparing for Transplant	53
Chapter 13	The Call	57
Chapter 14	Post-Transplant Challenges	61
Chapter 15	Post-Transplant Recuperation	67
Chapter 16	Long-Awaited Make-A-Wish	71
Chapter 17	Chilling Experiences	75
Chapter 18	Chicken Pox	79
Chapter 19	Additional Health Issues	85
Chapter 20	A Year Following Transplant	87

Chapter 21	Many Additional Medical Problems Cropping Up	89
Chapter 22	Struggling to Start Life Over	95
Chapter 23	A Thick Black Veil Falls	101
Chapter 24	Processing the Grief	105
Chapter 25	Difficulty Letting Go	109
Chapter 26	Slogging Through the Darkness, Searching for Any Fragment of Light	113
Chapter 27	A Child in Spirit ~	117
Chapter 28	Thank You	121
Chapter 29	Love Echoes	123
Chapter 30	"Ode to Josh"	125
Chapter 31	"Why Does It Happen?"	135
Chapter 32	"The Dragon Asked"	137
Appendix A	Organs for Transplant	139
Appendix B	Tissues for Transplant	143
Appendix C	Donation Myths	145
Appendix D	Living Donation	147
Appendix E	Support Organizations	153
Appendix F	Further Reading	155

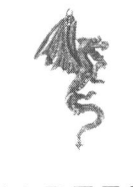

CHAPTER 1

A New Little Person

I was introduced to Josh Allan Mickelson on Saturday, November 28, 1981. A true gift from God, he was a teacher in his own right, a kind, gentle old spirit. He came to teach humility, perseverance, compassion, determination, unconditional love and most of all, strength of character to those whose lives he touched. How could I possibly ignore this generous gift and fail to take advantage of the golden opportunity I had just received? Life had suddenly, irreversibly, become *not about me*.

The marvel of this most precious child's birth is a story of its own. My water broke on Thursday, Thanksgiving evening and on Friday evening my OB/GYN physician instructed me to proceed to the hospital to be examined. I was then admitted to the hospital, and our long journey began.

When it was determined late Friday night that a Caesarian Section delivery would be necessary, my doctor would need to locate the only OB/GYN surgeon in town. As luck would have it, that lone surgeon had recently lost his partner and he himself was out of town for the holiday. The only general surgeon in Warren was also out of town and unavailable. She finally resorted to calling in a retired surgeon to do my C-Section.

Lying on an OR table early Saturday morning, I felt someone scrubbing my belly with betadine. I clearly recall being terrified that the surgeon would begin to use the scalpel while I was still awake; I tightly grasped his hand and heard him comment to the nurses about this. It turned out that this surgeon had never used the low transverse incision, so I was split from stem to stern, so to speak, my bikini days a thing of the past. I recognize now that this thought was so very ego-driven. This concern and my ego quickly fell off the priority list. My primary worry was for a critically ill baby struggling to cling to life.

Still groggy and recovering in the Critical Care Unit (there being no Recovery Room staffing on Saturdays), my own OB/GYN physician arrived and said, "There's a problem." Even in my medicated state of mind, I realized that this was alarming statement, prophetic of impending trials and heartaches to come. The doctor explained to me that my baby was having difficulty breathing and plans were in the works to have him transferred as soon as possible to Buffalo Children's Hospital. I slipped back into my drug-induced haze, remembering little more about the time immediately following Josh's birth.

Josh's pediatrician later explained to me that as soon as Josh was born, he was a nice healthy pink color. But he quickly became blue, then "pinked up" once more with oxygen, but his oxygen saturation ("sats") again rapidly dropped off.[2] True to his vibrant spirit, he was a colorful child even then.

Josh was quickly whisked away from the operating room to the nursery, where an intravenous (IV) line was initiated in the umbilical vein, a nasogastric (NG)[3] tube inserted, a catheter was introduced into his bladder, a pulse oximeter[4] placed on a finger, and last but certainly not least, he was intubated[5] so a ventilator could effectively breathe for him. Tachypnea[6] was one of his symptoms; aspiration of amniotic fluid was suspected.

Later, in the early afternoon, the Buffalo Children's Hospital (BCH) ambulance crew arrived to transport Josh. They brought him to my bedside

---

[2] . Sometimes referred to as O sats, or simply, sats. Refers to the extent to which hemoglobin is saturated with oxygen. Normal oxygen saturation is usually between 96 percent and 98 percent. - verywellhealth

[3] . A tube that is passed through the nose and down through the nasopharynx and esophagus into the stomach. It is a flexible tube made of rubber or plastic, and it has bidirectional potential. - MedicineNet

[4] . A device that measures the oxygen saturation of arterial blood in a subject by utilizing a sensor attached typically to a finger, toe, or ear to determine the percentage of oxyhemoglobin in blood pulsating through a network of capillaries. - Merriam-Webster

[5] . The process of inserting a tube through the mouth and then into the airway. This is done so that a patient can be placed on a ventilator to assist with breathing during anesthesia, sedation, or severe illness. - verywellhealth

[6] . An elevated respiratory rate, or more simply, breathing that is more rapid than normal. - verywellhealth

and kindly asked if I would like to tell him goodbye, as they needed to leave for Buffalo immediately. I strained to partially sit up and patted him, taking in his pretty little face and tiny body surrounded by all those medical devices necessary to keep him alive. I was left with only three blurry, dark, poor-quality Polaroid pictures of his naked little body to comfort me through the next two desolate weeks.

In Buffalo it was found that Josh had significant gastroesophageal reflux (GERD) with aspiration.[7] During the months following my surgery and the birth of my child, I slowly gathered my wits about me. Recalling the meeting just a few short months before with Josh's pediatrician, we discussed the now comparatively simple process of circumcision. This trivial procedure had now totally dropped off our priority list due to Josh's unremitting struggle for survival. In reflection, how far from our thoughts this decision was in our precious child's life. I never dreamed that we would be praying for his very next breath.

Due to the transverse (classical) incision technique used for his C-Section delivery I was not permitted to travel for two weeks. At this point, this was a harrowing time for me not being able to see my baby. Jan went to Buffalo to visit on the following weekend with his mother, June.

Concerned friends would ask Josh's birth weight, but at the time the situation was so critical immediately following birth, I wasn't even sure what his weight was. I learned later that his weight was 7 pounds, which is not a low birth weight. The physicians estimated that he was born about a month early. Initially the doctors suspected meconium aspiration syndrome (MAS) as the culprit of Josh's respiratory distress.[8] Later their thoughts were more focused on cystic fibrosis (CF).[9]

---

[7] . Gastroesophageal reflux disease, or GERD, is a digestive disorder that affects the lower esophageal sphincter (LES), the ring of muscle between the esophagus and stomach. Many people, including pregnant women, suffer from heartburn or acid indigestion caused by GERD. - WebMD

[8] . Meconium aspiration syndrome is trouble breathing (respiratory distress) in a newborn who has breathed (aspirated) a dark green, sterile fecal material called meconium into the lungs before or around the time of birth. - Merck Manual

[9] . Cystic fibrosis is a progressive, genetic disease that causes persistent lung infections and limits the ability to breathe over time. In people with CF, a defective gene causes a thick, sticky buildup of mucus in the lungs, pancreas, and other organs. - Cystic Fibrosis Foundation

Homebound, I designed and maintained my own copies of Josh's growth, weight and meal charts to somehow construct a tangible attachment, a fragile, invisible filament connecting me to my distant baby. My charts contained his weight, length, amounts of feedings, every prized morsel of information the nurses would provide for me on a daily basis. It occurred to me at this point that Josh may not survive this horrifying ordeal.

Those first two weeks alone at home were interminable for me. I was isolated, depressed and in pure emotional and mental misery. Developing and maintaining the charts helped me to pass the time and distract me from the reality of the situation, the inconceivable possibility of the loss of our baby. It felt incredibly strange realizing I might not even recognize my own baby as I had only a few minutes with him before the BCH staff whisked him away.

Finally permitted to travel, the one-and-a-half-hour trip to Buffalo in a snowy December seemed endless. If anyone ever requested an actual "beam me up", it was me. Where was Star Trek technology when you needed it? The weekend trips over the next months seemed never-ending, not to mention this was the worst time of year for the weather in northwestern Pennsylvania and western New York. Somewhere in the flats between Sinclairville and Cassadaga, New York, snow blew horizontally across the road in front of us, resulting in whiteouts and vast white drifts across fields and roads. This created a painfully slow trip, not to mention abundant tension in my gut; would we ever get there? A normally one-and-a-half-hour drive easily turned into a two-and-a-half to three-hour trip, enormously nerve wracking and decidedly stressful as it was robbing us of treasured time with our son.

I remember feeling incredibly anxious on my initial visit to the Buffalo Children's Hospital Neonatal Intensive Care Unit (NICU) when Josh was two weeks old.[10] At thirty-one years of age I had never cared for a baby; child care was a totally foreign concept to me. I came to the sudden realization that I didn't know how to be a mother. My future was on the threshold of changing forever.

So here we were, Jan and I, thrust into the glaring lights of the NICU, never suspecting this would be the center of our world for months to

---

[10] . Newborn, or Neonatal, Intensive Care Unit, an intensive care unit designed for premature and ill newborn babies. - MedicineNet

come. We found ourselves listening to instructions for hand scrubbing and gowning before we were permitted to enter the clean environment. A cold? Masking and hand scrubbing unquestionably were a necessity to protect all the little ones in the unit.

We were led past seemingly endless isolettes filled with critically ill infants, some crying, some peacefully resting in their little transparent enclosures. I sensed that there may be some who were destined to never see their homes; I prayed I was wrong. On the bad days, and we certainly had plenty of those, I prayed that our own baby would not be one of those.

The nurse directed us to Josh's isolette. He was lying there naked except for a tiny diaper, utterly helpless in his little environment, on oxygen, an IV in a tiny vein, an NG tube used for all his feedings. His little chest was retracting alarmingly.[11] I was near panicking, but trusted the nurses would be aware of any problems. Wouldn't they?

A gloomy cloud of dread hovered over me every waking moment during those first months. Between these moments, fleetingly, I realized how fortunate we were even to have a surviving baby. I reminded myself to be grateful and to try to stay positive, a difficult task at best. On the good days, I rejoiced in the newness of being a mother, those gorgeous blue eyes looking innocently up at me as I rocked, hummed, smiled and talked to him. "I'm your mama, little one." I wondered what he was thinking about this strange, bright and noisy environment he had been thrust into.

The huge NICU held 30 or 40 babies and was filled with noise; beeping monitors, flashing lights, blaring alarms, whirring machines, crying, and anxious parents in rockers murmuring to their precious little ones. There was the unvarying sound of nurse's voices, calling to each other for assistance, speaking softly to their tiny charges, giving advice and reassuring frightened parents like ourselves. Frightened? Perhaps 'terrified' is a much more honest and accurate adjective.

The nurses were in perpetual motion, flitting from patient to patient, constantly washing their sore, dry and cracked hands. They were responsible for so many tiny lives in their care. God bless them for choosing this profession. Much later when I found time to actually think rationally

---

[11] . A retraction is a medical term for when the area between the ribs and in the neck sinks in when a person with asthma attempts to inhale. Retractions are a sign someone is working hard to breathe. ... But if a person is having trouble breathing, extra muscles kick into action. - KidsHealth

about this extraordinary journey, I recognized how demanding their job was. I found myself pondering how difficult yet wonderful it was for them when a baby finally got to go home. I couldn't—no, *I wouldn't*—consider any different outcome for us.

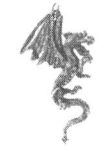

CHAPTER 2

Watching Josh Improve

Jan and I were in a continual panicked and helpless state, watching our tiny child fight just to draw his next breath. I had been encouraged to pump my breasts and freeze the milk to feed him on the weekends. Josh was experiencing chest retractions forgoing any attempt for me to breast feed. His breathing was an absolute priority. He took very little formula and constantly struggled to gain weight.

We would take a break to have lunch and visit the hospital gift shop. On one such visit we saw a stuffed animal there that made us think of Josh – a camel with his legs tucked under him, head tilted to the side, eyes closed, snoozing. The camel was dubbed Omar and promptly took his place on top of Josh's isolette, dutifully watching over him. Unfortunately, several weeks later Omar went to stuffed animal heaven as a ceiling leak had rendered him unsanitary. So next we found a colorful macaw, and since a guy couldn't have a "Polly" parrot, we dubbed him "Paul". Later we added Klondike a big, tan cuddly soft bear from somewhere far up north. He was just perfect for hugging. Paul now perches near my computer and reminds me of long-ago days when life was a challenge. Seeing Paul here with me brings joy, remembering that at the time when he was new, this beautiful child was alive and fighting his courageous battle.

The NICU nurse would let us know when it was time to feed Josh. Holding the feeding syringe that was attached to his NG tube, we would slightly elevate it to allow a few cc's of formula to drip slowly into his stomach. Josh's hyperinflated lungs were compressing his stomach which allowed very little space for vital nutrition. To this day I recall the grip of fear that this scene brought to me. Inside his isolette on oxygen, Josh was invariably sitting in a partially upright position in his "Easy Babe" seat. This was to prevent aspiration of his formula and to help control the constant gastroesophageal reflux and aspiration of stomach acid.[12]

At this point, with more than 11 years' hospital experience, I had effectively learned to remove my personal feelings while working in the Medical Imaging field. This however, was an unequaled, particularly strange and tremendously distressing experience. It is unquestionably an entirely different matter when it's about the very life of your own child, making it absolutely impossible, at least for me, to step back and detach.

We were driving home one dark and dreary Sunday evening from Buffalo on Route 90 which runs parallel to Lake Erie. The lake-effect snow was so wet and heavy that it stuck to the headlights requiring us to pull over several times to wipe them clean. People were pulled off the road everywhere. Were we insane to be traveling in this weather? Surely God watched over us every weekend as we traveled back and forth in this winters' miserable weather conditions, to where our precious child lay, sometimes just barely clinging to life.

Unbeknownst to me, Josh and I must have bonded sometime between minute one and minute two of our first meeting. In retrospect, perhaps it truly occurred months prior to actually seeing each other face-to-face; perhaps it was more of a face-to-belly knowing. In spite of this, because of my inexperience with babies and children, it felt very awkward the first time I held him. It was made even more challenging by holding the corrugated aerosol tubing close to his face and being very cautious not to inadvertently tug on his NG tube. It soon became comfortable to hold, comfort and rock him, looking into his searching eyes. He had finally found Mom and Dad in this loud, bright and distracting place.

Other firsts were just as delightfully extraordinary: changing his little diaper, putting on a t-shirt, bathing him in a basin. I have a great Polaroid of him sitting in a wash basin, looking at me out of the corner of his eye, appearing to have a smirk on his face. I wondered, "Do you know I'm Mom?" Now, the response I hear deep in my soul is, "Sure I did, Mom!"

---

[12] . Pulmonary aspiration is when you inhale food, stomach acid, or saliva into your lungs. - WebMD

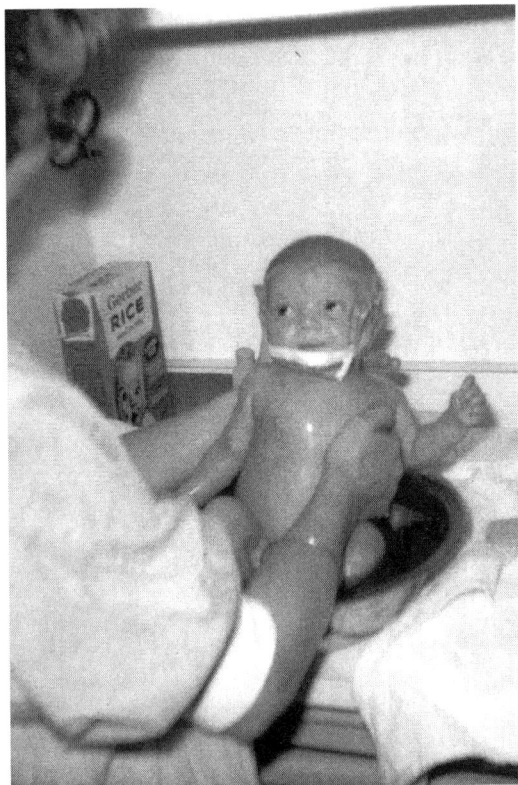

Josh (age 2 months) and his first "Mom bath".

We were especially grateful for use of the Parents Room at the hospital, a small cramped room with bunk beds and a rocker where we could rest, sleep and shower, returning refreshed to visit Josh again. When that was unavailable, the conference room with fold-down chairs doubled as our bedroom. The staff was very compassionate with the highly stressed parents of their tiny patients.

On our way to scrubbing our hands and donning clean long-sleeve yellow gowns each time, we walked down the hallway toward the NICU after checking in at the nurse's desk. There were photo boards filled with wonderful pictures of smiling babies who had happily gone home. This possibility was a remote concept to us when Josh was only two weeks old. The first couple weeks I painfully glanced at the photos of former NICU occupants that proud parents had sent. Soon I learned to avert my eyes to avoid the unpleasant aching in my heart. We weren't yet able to see that light at the end of our tunnel. I recall strong feelings of guilt for my envy of what those photos represented. Months later I was finally able to fully appreciate that parents wanted the nurses to see their beautiful, now healthy children. However, at the time it was so difficult as we were forced to acknowledge that we were nowhere near that point in our child's life.

At this stressful time, joy appeared to be beyond our visible horizons. We were on our own private convoluted path and found that we would be required to travel through prolonged sadness in order to come out the other side into the sunshine. It was almost as if we had to demonstrate ourselves worthy of his life and his love. Nothing builds an appreciation for a beloved child's life like a chronic, life-threatening disease.

Very early on, the doctors told us they suspected that Josh had aspirated amniotic fluid or meconium. Although he weighed seven pounds and was born on his predicted due date, we eventually learned that he was in actuality about four or five weeks premature. In premature infants the lungs are known to be underdeveloped. Any or all of these factors could have been responsible for his current status. It looked to us as though he was hanging on by a thread—or perhaps more accurately, by many tubes.

My mother and my stepfather, Chuck, had postponed their routine winter departure for Florida until after Josh's birth. They finally left in January when it became clear that he would not be coming home soon. After 6 weeks, I had been cleared to return to work and I did so with enthusiasm. This was a great distraction from the unrelenting anxiety and helplessness of having our critically ill infant so far away from us. I desperately needed to focus on something besides the pain and discomfort that Josh was in.

When Jan and I arrived at the hospital the weekend of Valentine's Day 1982, Josh was sitting up in his Easy Babe seat. He was sealed inside a tiny clear plastic oxygen tent on 100% oxygen, struggling for each breath, experiencing chest retractions. This was when my greatest fears finally bubbled up into awareness, no longer to be denied. I was terrified that this treasured little person was close to leaving us but dared not put it into words. We stood beside him crying, unable to hold or touch him to assure him that we were there. Desperate, I silently prayed, "Please God, don't take our precious, beautiful child."

Looking through my tears at his pretty little face with bluish lips, I continued to speak silently, directly to the only one who could help. I remember thinking, "Please, God, let him live and don't let him be brain damaged." As I glanced over at the two-and-one-half pound little girl in the isolette next to him I thought, "If that tiny little girl can make it in this world, please let our baby survive." It was so difficult leaving that weekend; it seemed that my heart would burst with pain. The intense ache and feeling of absolute hopelessness were unbearable. This was a seemingly endless period filled with anxiety and depression contrasted by hope, prayer and a new-found love.

The next weekend, it was shocking to find that Josh had been placed on a ventilator. The endotracheal tube was holding his vocal cords open but I could see that Josh was crying silently.[13] During a previous visit, I had helped to hold him still for drawing of Arterial Blood Gases from an artery in his wrist. This time I held him tightly for the insertion of a scalp vein needle. These were all a part of our enormous apparently never-ending nightmare, but I knew I had to be there with him and for him.

"Please God, let it be me instead" must be every parent's plea under similar circumstances. Much later I was to realize that this was only the first of many identical prayers. Upon reflection, I recognize that we dug down deep inside and somewhere found the strength to endure each unbearable ordeal with this beautiful child. I suspect I dominated a lot of God's time with all my selfish pleas.

It seemed that almost every weekend when we arrived to visit Josh he was in a different location in the NICU. Initially it was a shock to look in the space where he was last week to find another baby, terrifying thoughts instantly flooding in. We quickly came to learn that isolette moves were a common occurrence in the NICU setting.

I called the nurses every weekday to check on Josh's status. I was consumed with maintaining charts of his length, weight and formula quantity to track his progress. In the beginning, when I would phone each Friday, I asked whether we should bring the car seat that weekend—was he ready to be discharged? I posed this question only for the first six weeks because the answer always led to the same disappointment. We were continuously living in the realm of the unknown.

Friends continued to ask how much he had weighed when he was born. I didn't verbalize this, but thought, "He's alive…what else is important?" I realized they had only asked because they cared. I couldn't find records

---

[13] . A small usually plastic tube inserted into the trachea through the mouth or nose to maintain an unobstructed passageway especially to deliver oxygen or anesthesia to the lungs - called also breathing tube. - Merriam-Webster Medical

that documented his weight at birth, which is reasonable, considering the on-going life-saving measures that were being utilized. Later I learned from the NICU that he had weighed 7 pounds upon arrival. At that time, every other statistic was insignificant; the only important detail was that our child remained alive.

In February 1982, Josh developed Respiratory Syncytial Virus infection (RSV)[14]. RSV is very contagious and much like a bad cold, causes all the same signs and symptoms and is very common. Due to the risk of infection to the other neonates, Josh at the age of three months, was transferred to a private room on a different floor. As impossible and distressing as it was to us, he was without the comforting, constant watchful nursing care that existed in the NICU. Learning of this transfer immediately triggered profound anxiety in us.

In retrospect this was a traumatic but promising occasion. The doctors must have decided that Josh was well enough to be moved to his own room. This had to be a good sign. He weighed about eight pounds by then and was actually in a crib, though still in his Easy Babe seat and on oxygen. At the time, the switch to a crib seemed a tangible upgrade in his progress. OK, I conceded that there might be a light at the end of this seemingly unending, twisted tunnel.

Test results were negative when checking for allergies Alpha-1 Antitrypsin Deficiency[15] and multiple sweat tests for Cystic Fibrosis (CF). Josh, at three months of age, underwent an open-lung biopsy to determine precisely what was causing his constant respiratory distress.[16] Waiting anxiously in the surgical waiting room, we could not bring ourselves to leave for lunch for fear that the doctor would come out to bring us an update about Josh's surgery. We had been told that someone would come to the waiting room after the surgery had been completed to discuss how it

---

[14] . Respiratory Syncytial Virus (RSV) is a common, and very contagious, virus that infects the respiratory tract of most children before their second birthday. - WebMD

[15] . Alpha-1 Antitrypsin Deficiency (A1AD) is a hereditary disorder characterized by low levels of a protein called alpha-1 antitrypsin (A1AT) which is found in the blood. - WebMD

[16] . A sweat test measures the amount of salt chemicals (sodium and chloride) in sweat. It is done to help diagnose cystic fibrosis. Normally, sweat on the skin surface contains very little sodium and chloride. People with cystic fibrosis have 2 to 5 times the normal amount of sodium and chloride in their sweat. - WebMD

had gone. We sat with other parents in the waiting room, seeing them leave one by one, waiting seemingly an eternity to hear some news. I became increasingly concerned with each passing minute. As it was taking much longer than we had originally been advised, I repeatedly checked at the desk with the volunteer and finally, actually dreading to hear the response, requested again that she check on his status. We at last learned that Josh had been returned to ICU two hours before. Distraught that we had been unnecessarily delayed, we hurried away to find our son.

This was the conscious beginning of a learning process for me about being your loved one's advocate. When necessary, you must courteously but firmly insist that information be supplied. There is no one who will care more than you.

When we were finally permitted into the Recovery Room to see Josh, we could not hold or even touch him for fear of stimulating and triggering him to cry even more. How helpless, isolated and out of my element I felt, tears streaming down my face. Josh was crying and clearly in distress. Was he in pain? We were asked to leave to allow the staff uninterrupted time and space to do their important work. It was such a desolate feeling, not knowing his medical status, unable to touch, hold or comfort him.

A few days later we finally received the diagnosis, established through the open-lung biopsy. It was a very strange medical term: Desquamative Interstitial Pneumonitis [or Desquamative Interstitial Pneumonia] (DIP).[17] Over time we became very familiar with the diagnosis. Throughout Josh's life it became increasingly apparent that many physicians we came in contact with knew very little about this rare form of interstitial lung disease.[18]

A Pulmonologist at Children's Hospital of Pittsburgh (CHP) stated in a letter to Josh's pediatrician in March of 1982 that DIP was being more frequently described in children. It was typically a pathologic diagnosis, usually secondary to some underlying "insult". In Josh's case that insult was probably the pneumonitis that he had experienced in his first couple days of life.

---

[17] . Desquamative interstitial pneumonia is a type of idiopathic interstitial pneumonia. The vast majority of adult patients with desquamative interstitial pneumonia are smokers, who tend to develop the disease in their 30s or 40s. - MERCK MANUAL-Professional Version

[18] . Interstitial lung disease describes a large group of disorders, most of which cause progressive scarring of lung tissue. - Mayo Clinic

Josh's stomach was being compressed by his hyperinflated lungs and could hold only small amounts of formula. His labored breathing was burning more calories than he could take in. Struggling throughout his life to thrive, gain weight and grow, every ounce gained was precious and hard-earned. Josh consistently remained at or below the lowest curve of the growth chart for his age group.

CHAPTER 3

A Smile!

We saw Josh's first smile when he was about three and a half months of age. What a delight this was and an extraordinarily mood-lifting sight. I have a great Polaroid of this special moment that we experienced. At the time I wondered who was the first to see this gorgeous smile. What else were we missing each day as he grew older?

This occasion reminded me that while Josh was still a patient in the NICU there was a little girl, 18 months old, who was finally going home. A year and a half! It was difficult to imagine this situation and I prayed that this would not be the case with Josh. There I go again, begging God for mercy for this little boy. It was so exciting although intimidating to lose that support when bringing an ill child home from the hospital. I now realize how important it was simply to be grateful that Josh came home at all. Thank you, thank you, thank you, God!

On March 20, 1982, we received the exciting news—Josh was finally coming home the next weekend! He would be just four months old when he finally came out into the big world. In preparation, Josh must be weaned off oxygen while maintaining an acceptable oxygen saturation level while on room air over the next seven days. That meant that without oxygen therapy, his oxygen blood level must remain in the 95–100 percent range.

Josh's lungs were hyperinflated, caused by the air trapping characteristic of DIP, his chronic lung disease. [19] There was abnormal retention of air in the constricted lower airways of the lungs following expiration, making it difficult for him to productively cough to move the mucus up and out of his lungs. As he grew older, this trapping of air produced a gradual chest deformity to develop, called pectus carinatum, a protrusion of the sternum and ribs. This protrusion became increasingly more apparent as time went on and the disease progressed.

Arriving at BCH on a Saturday morning, March 27th, we were instructed on the essential timing of medications and their safe sequencing between meals and breathing treatments. We learned proper and specific positioning, taking advantage of gravity using postural drainage (PD)[20] in combination with chest percussions.[21] This was a fairly complicated procedure for us to learn and in the beginning, after only a few minutes of this process, my elbows and wrists began to ache. We used towels or blankets to appropriately position Josh's body and initially we constantly referred to the positioning diagrams we were provided.

The above described Chest Physiotherapy (CPT) is a technique that uses the vibrations from chest percussions to loosen and move secretions in the lower airways into larger ones where it can be more easily moved out by coughing.[22] Each position clears a different lobe of the lungs and positioning is dependent upon which lobe of the lung is being treated. The

---

[19] . Hyperinflated lungs occur when air gets trapped in the lungs and causes them to overinflate. ... Hyperinflated lungs are often seen in people with chronic obstructive pulmonary disease (COPD) — a disorder that includes emphysema. Certain lung problems, such as asthma and cystic fibrosis, also can cause hyperinflation. – Mayo Clinic

[20] . A therapy for clearing congested lungs by placing the patient in a position for drainage by gravity, often accompanied by percussion with hollowed hands. – Dictionary.com

[21] . Chest percussion (chest physiotherapy) uses clapping of the chest with a cupped hand to vibrate the airways in the lungs. This vibration moves the mucus from smaller airways into larger ones where it can be coughed up. Chest percussion is done with the help of a partner, special electronic devices designed to vibrate the chest, or other instruments that a person can use to vibrate the chest safely. - www.uofmhealth.org

[22] . Chest physiotherapy (CPT) is the treatment generally performed by physical therapists and respiratory therapists, whereby breathing is improved by the indirect removal of mucus from the breathing passages of a patient - Wikipedia.

patient is positioned on the back, stomach or side, partially turned with the upper or lower torso elevated. This airway clearing technique is utilized on those who have lung conditions, such as DIP or Cystic Fibrosis, that make it difficult to clear mucus from the lungs. The risk of lung infection increases when mucus collects in the lungs, so this is a crucial practice for some patients.

As unpleasant as the postural drainage and chest percussion procedure seems for the patient, it was one vital phase in the on-going treatment of Josh's disease. This treatment was required four times a day following each of his breathing treatments.[23] The breathing treatments made use of a mini air compressor along with a nebulizer and medications intended to open airways. It was remarkable to watch Josh tolerate this entire process, his little body bouncing from the vigorous percussions. He seemingly took it all in stride, a normal part of his day and his life.

Is spite of all this going on in our lives, suddenly colors seemed to deepen, the sun shone brighter and birds began to sing again. I hadn't realized how I had essentially shut down to the everyday, wonderful occurrences around us. Josh was finally home!

As organization seems to be my forte, I created an 8½" x 11" notebook page completely filled (yes, literally) with scheduled times for all our tasks. This was to enable me to systematically establish the sequencing of all the daily required tasks. Bronkosol and Intal Inhalation (breathing treatment medications) was regularly scheduled four times throughout the day. Meals had to be given at least two hours before treatments so no vomiting or aspiration would occur. If the liquid oral Theophylline (Slo-Phyllin), a medication given every six hours, was spit up or choked on, we had to estimate how much Josh got, and re-administer the remainder. The pressure was at an extreme level, adrenaline constantly giving me a burst of energy. It was next to impossible to sleep.

Theophylline is a drug utilized to prevent and treat wheezing, shortness of breath, and chest tightness caused by asthma, chronic bronchitis, emphysema and other lung diseases. It relaxes and opens air passages in the lungs, making it easier for the patient to breathe. Prednisone was initially

---

[23] . A nebulizer is an electrically powered machine that turns liquid medication into a mist so that it can be breathed directly into the lungs through a face mask or mouthpiece. People with asthma can use a nebulizer to take their medications. – KidsHealth

prescribed for Josh every other day; as a result, we had to be concerned about his eye health and an eye exam was required every six months to remain alert for cataracts.

After coming home, Josh spent twenty-four hours a day sitting up in an Easy-Babe seat, as he had during his entire four-month hospital stay. It was incredibly tense for a couple weeks until I was able to establish a routine that eventually flowed efficiently. His first meal at home was a half-ounce of formula. I panicked and feared he would starve to death on my watch. Scary? Absolutely alarming!

Naturally family and friends were anxious to meet Josh, but we needed to be cautious about exposing him to respiratory and other infections, so visits at first were short, if not non-existent. Upon return from the Sunshine State in April, Mom saw the difficulty we had struggling with Josh for his PD (postural drainage) positioning. With Chuck's help, she designed and built an angled board to help simplify positioning for chest percussions. Mom really was born before her time and should have been an engineer.

On a happier note, our two Scottish Terriers, Lady Macbeth (Mac) and Sally Jo had been waiting anxiously at home to meet their new brother. As Josh grew older and was able to get around in his little walker, he came to love these dogs dearly. The sister-dogs reciprocated and were so gentle with him. Josh would stand on a hassock to peer out the front picture window. There was just enough room for one of the dogs to stand beside him. With paws on the windowsill they helped to scrutinize and direct whatever fascinating activity might be occurring out there. When Josh was older, he would help shampoo and brush Mac and Sally Jo and loved them up all the time. What great sisters they were!

Much to my surprise, gradually over the next several months caring for Josh became easier as we established our routine. We began to relax a little and have delightfully fun times. I vividly recall the time I tiptoed into his bedroom to check on him while he was napping and found him standing, reaching out from his crib pulling tissues out of a box. They were all over him and the floor, and he was smiling his bright, beautiful smile at me. What a memorable picture that made!

Josh and I spent lots of time outside that summer of 1982. We took walks with Mac and Sally Jo in the woods behind our house. As I mowed,

I carried him in a backpack, secure and often snoozing. I guess I have myself to blame, as this probably began his lifelong love of lawn mowers, weed whips, four-wheelers, motorcycles, snowmobiles and a generous assortment of other noisy, motorized equipment.

CHAPTER 4

Hospital Admissions

Late April 1982 brought a frightening hospital admission. Josh, 5 months of age, had an increased respiratory rate and chest retractions. Because we were so familiar with his PD and Chest Physical Therapy (CPT), I was asked to do these treatments following his breathing treatments. He was diagnosed with viral pneumonitis and was an inpatient for three days while being started on an antibiotic.

Two months later, near the end of June, Josh was again admitted to Warren General Hospital for a rash and acute respiratory distress with wheezing, rales and retractions noted, a probable viral illness to blame. Antibiotics were again prescribed, with continuation of his chronic medications and treatments. He was discharged the next day, wheezing and retractions having cleared.

I was grateful for the quick recovery, given how worried I was during these illnesses and hospital admissions. It was a huge relief to have Josh back home where I could monitor him 24/7.

In July that year, my dear gentle grandmother lost her battle with diabetes and heart disease. Following her funeral in Erie, Pennsylvania, when it was time for Josh's breathing treatment and PD, a relative commented, "What a good mother you are, doing all those treatments." That was an absurd concept to me then and seemed to me a task not much more than feeding, bathing and all the other tasks that a parent would normally perform in the daily care of their child. It was all in a day's work and a vital part of our daily routine. Under these circumstances I knew that any parent would do the same. We simply had additional responsibilities and deeply appreciated the bright light Josh had brought into our lives. This was made easier as we were acutely aware that his fragile state of health and happiness could change at any moment.

August that same year brought an ER visit due to an increased respiratory rate, rales and wheezing, which ended in discharge with merely a medication adjustment. Whew, we dodged the bullet on that one!

As a result of a BCH Lung Center visit, Josh at 10 months of age, was finally was old enough to use Theodur sprinkles, a twelve-hour time-release Theophylline dose he could take with applesauce. At that point, our lives improved significantly and we all could all get a full night's sleep. During our visit, the Pulmonologist suggested smaller and more frequent meals, discouraging cereals and vegetables since they had such low caloric content. He also suggested that we augment Josh's diet with ENSURE Plus as well as adding corn oil to his formula for the extra caloric value to his intake.

A dear friend was thrilled to care for Josh, so I went back to work after spending a wonderful six-month leave together. We lived contentedly day-to-day, watching Josh grow emotionally and mentally but very little physically. We had regularly scheduled appointments with Dr. Gerd Cropp, the pulmonologist at the Buffalo Children's Hospital Lung Clinic. Josh would have further sweat tests, again, to rule out Cystic Fibrosis. In addition to this were skin (allergy) testing, Nuclear Medicine Ventilation and Perfusion Lung Scans, routine chest x-rays and Pulmonary Function Testing (PFT). Lab testing was also done to check for appropriate medication levels.[24] He continued to use so many calories struggling to breathe that he was able to gain little ground on the weight and growth chart.

At one of our many outpatient visits, one of the BCH Pulmonologists noted that Josh was beginning to exhibit clubbing of his fingers. Clubbing often occurs in patients with heart and lung diseases, which reduce the amount of oxygen in the blood. These diseases include lung disorders in which the deep lung tissues become swollen and then scarred, e.g., interstitial lung disease, with which Josh had been diagnosed. A common indication of clubbing, which I had begun to notice, was that the last part of the finger may appear large or bulging and the nail curves downward so it looks like the rounded part of an upside-down spoon.

---

[24] . Lung function tests check how well your lungs work. The tests can find lung problems, measure how serious they are, and check to see how well treatment for a lung disease is working. - WebMD

We were told early in Josh's life that a lung transplant might well be in his future. Transplant? What a foreign concept this was to us in the early 1980's. I was quite confident that this extreme treatment would never be required for my son. Transplant? No, not us! That chilling possibility was filed away until a much later date when it could no longer be denied.

Josh continued to have chest x-rays, PFTs and Lung Scans on a regular basis. During the many trips to the Buffalo Children's Hospital (BCH) Lung Center for checkups, I took some opportunities to privately point out to Josh how very fortunate he was that he was merely short of breath. Wasn't he lucky? He could run and play, but that little boy was in a reclining wheelchair and could not even hold his head up. There were so many heart-breaking sights to be observed if only you were able to see past your own heart-rending challenges. God Bless all parents of the health-challenged children we encountered during our many hospital visits. I was always aware that we were so very fortunate that this was the only challenge Josh faced, trying to instill in him gratitude for what health he did have, a difficult lesson for his mom.

CHAPTER 5

Let the Fun Begin!

It's interesting and comical how children hear certain things differently and adapt them to terms they understand. Josh loved to watch Indiana Jones movies and called one of them, "Raiders of the Lost *Dark*" and a character in another movie was "Dark Vader". The thing that flies in the wind at airports was called a "wind socket". So funny! I wish I had recorded so many of the wonderful mind-creations that I'd heard. He loved the Little Critter books when he was little, and at the age of two, could remember every word of a fire engine book we read every night.

One day when he was about two years old, I asked, "Josh, what's your middle name?" To my delight, his honest and innocent two-year old reply was "Ua." Josh-Ua? Although his given name was Josh, we found that people sometimes would just automatically add the "Ua" and he had learned the extension through them. Another lesson I added to my gratitude inventory: be appreciative for each little story and the amusing, although minor, events.

Josh and I went to Chapman Dam State Park for a picnic in the summer of 1984 to enjoy the sunshine, sand and water. We played at length on the beach, dripping wet sand into ever-growing sand castles around a temporary little lake we had carefully constructed. Over the years, hyperinflated lungs constantly pressed on his rib cage and sternum, gradually deforming the bones (pectus carinatum) thereby producing more room to accommodate his ever-expanding lungs.[25] A young boy about the age of seven walked past

---

[25] . Breastbone (sternum) and rib cartilage deformity that causes the chest to bow outward. It is caused by a defect in the tough connective tissue (cartilage) that holds the ribs to the breastbone. – Mayo Clinic

us on the beach and asked, "What's wrong with his chest?" Momentarily hesitating because I had never before been called upon for an explanation, I responded simply, "He was born with a lung disease." The boy looked a little shaken but I was struck by his short yet sympathetic response, "I'm sorry."

I began to realize that not everyone was going to be so empathetic or compassionate. Envisioning where he was on the growth chart in height and weight, I recognized that dealing with his disease he would always be very small for his age and a potential target for bullies. What a sad realization of the reality for my child.

We had enjoyed watching "The Karate Kid" numerous times and it was a theme that seemed to resonate with Josh. He began to imitate the moves of the Kata that Daniel was learning and was fascinated by the Japanese wisdom and tranquility imparted by Mr. Miyagi. I think intuitively he knew he would need that knowledge and strength of body and character in the future. I sensed that the karate moves he imitated needed some direction and focus.

So, shortly before his fourth birthday, Josh began a Shotokan Karate class. Martial Arts would also provide him with self-esteem and self-confidence, which would be essential due to his much smaller-than-average size. I knew he would to be the smallest in his class. I recognized that Josh may later need to utilize his martial arts skills for self-defense against bullies.

Rick Johnson was Josh's sensei (teacher) in Shotokan Karate and played a significant part in the moral person Josh became. He accepted Josh without question into the class despite his tender age and diminutive stature. I feel that Rick recognized that Josh needed direction and emotional support, perhaps sensing that this little boy was special in his own way. Many thanks to Rick for the patience, respect and understanding he showed Josh during the twelve years that he remained a devoted Karate student.

At four years old, he had begun attending Karate tournaments as a Yellow Belt and amazed some of the out-of-town sensei. They asked, "Who is that kid?" "Whose school is he with?" Josh had impressed many of them with the unusual moves he had created and frequently won trophies in the Mini-Mite class.

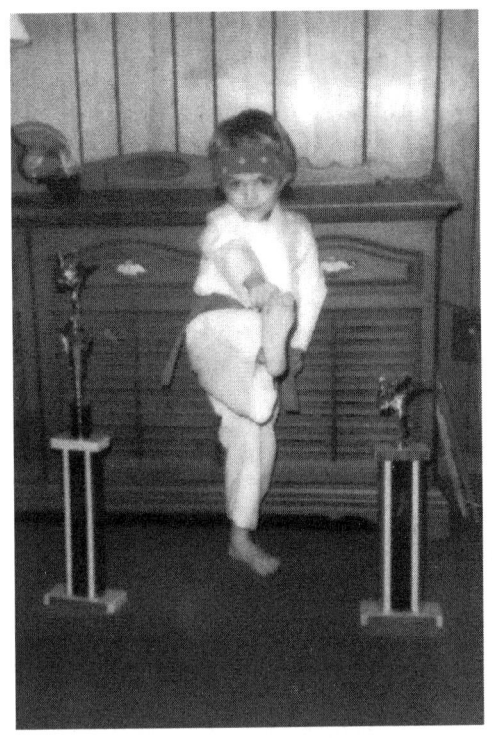

Josh (age 4, a blue belt) with his first trophies for early tournaments.

At one point Rick and I discussed the "free-form" kata Josh had created and used at tournaments. His kata changed with every presentation but nevertheless was winning trophies. We both recognized that as time went on judges would not permit this free-form technique and would hold him to his Shotokan roots.

When he was five Josh was congratulated by Sensei Rick Johnson at a local tournament for winning a trophy. Josh commented to Rick that he didn't *want* to win all the trophies. He wanted some of the other kids to win also. Coming from someone at such a young age, this comment completely floored me and my jaw dropped. This single statement embodied who Josh Allan Mickelson was and always would be.

I remember a competing student older than Josh who we frequently saw at tournaments. I noticed that Josh was irritated because he appeared cocky, loud, rude and offensive. Apparently, he had never learned how to lose gracefully. This student's parents would argue with the judges about his performance in front of him. Regardless of how it was earned, it appeared that he believed the award was the ultimate goal. I observed that this behavior offended and perplexed Josh even at this young age. How could I explain this behavior to him? His previous comment about winning took on an even deeper meaning, considering his reaction to this other boys' behavior.

Sensei Rick was understanding and compassionate with all his students. I firmly believed that we had made the right decision involving Josh in this training program. Because of his slight stature, I occasionally held up Rick as a positive example for Josh. Earning success and respect is in no way dependent upon a person's size or exterior appearance. The level of a person's integrity and what they carry in their heart is an integral part of one's accomplishments making that person larger than life.

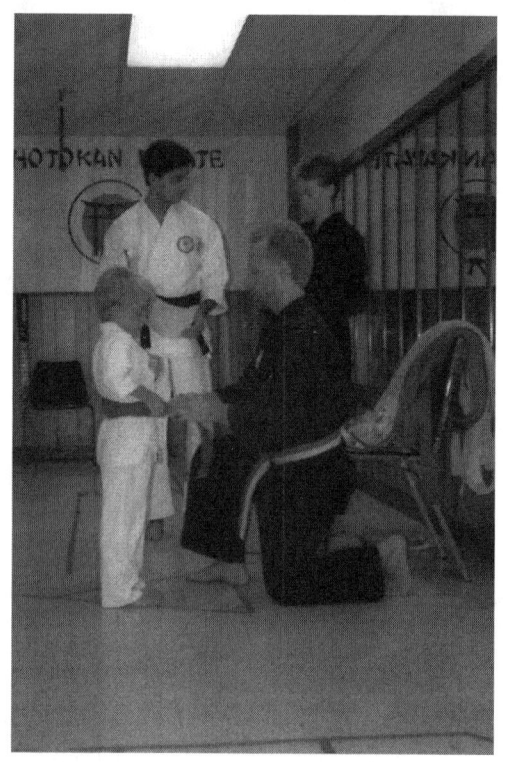

Josh, being awarded his purple belt

Josh's open and honest demeanor facilitated making friends and earned the respect of classmates and sensei's alike. He worked through the years steadily increasing his rank and eventually becoming a Black Belt. He was so proud when he finally earned the right to wear a hokama. A photo taken of him at this time shows how much pride he had in his hard-earned accomplishment.

CHAPTER 6

A Young Josh

On May 31, 1985, a tornado touched down nearby and a co-worker of Jan's sustained a serious head injury while unloading electric poles from a trailer, ultimately causing his death. Although Josh was only three and a half at the time, he developed a fear of thunderstorms because to him, it could also mean "tornado". His fear was that his dad or another loved one could be injured or worse. When Mom and I drove to Cambridge Springs one evening a couple years later, there were tornado warnings on the TV after we left. Josh and Chuck were fearful for our safety yet angry with us because we had driven through the storm and not called to assure them that all was well.

Mid-June of 1985 brought us another health scare, at age three. When I picked Josh up from the babysitter, he was lethargic, pale, feverish, vomiting and complaining of a severe headache. He was immediately admitted to the hospital with a fever, wheezing and retractions. Josh showed positive Brudzinski's Sign which could indicate meningitis.[26] Other possibilities mentioned were sepsis, Theophylline toxicity (there had been a recent adjustment of his dosage), viral illness or an electrolyte imbalance.[27]

---

[26] . One of the physically demonstrable symptoms of meningitis is Brudzinski's sign. Severe neck stiffness causes a patient's hips and knees to flex when the neck is flexed. – MedlinePlus

[27] . Sepsis is a potentially life-threatening complication of an infection. Sepsis occurs when chemicals released into the bloodstream to fight the infection trigger inflammatory responses throughout the body. This inflammation can trigger a cascade of changes that can damage multiple organ systems, causing them to fail. - Mayo Clinic

A spinal tap was performed in the ER prior to admission which was a terrifying procedure for both child and mom. Nauseated with worry, I did not want to lose this child. Much to my immense relief the results of his labwork and chest x-ray came back as negative and he was immediately started on an antibiotic. This was near the top of the list of the most frightening experiences we had had.

Another ER visit in November of the same year was necessary for left lower chest pain as well as an increased white count found on the lab tests. A chest x-ray comparison was made to multiple prior chest films but this time a left lower lobe pneumonia was found. A note in the reports made mention of Josh's chronic chest hyperinflation. Fortunately, no hospital admission was required, but an antibiotic was again prescribed.

When he was about four and a half years old, Dr. Cropp, BCH Pulmonologist, requested a Bone Age Study for Josh.[28] His chronologic age in April 1986 was almost four and a half years, but this x-ray revealed that he had a bone age of slightly over two and a half years, indicating significant bone growth delay. Due to his lung disease, his body burned calories much faster than normal, resulting in difficulty growing and thriving and he still remained well below normal on the growth chart for his age. In February, 1988, the Bone Age exam was repeated at age six years two months. The findings were consistent with a skeletal age of approximately four years nine months, at the very extreme limits of normal. This disease was keeping him small and struggling to maintain and gain weight.

In the fall of 1986, when Josh was almost five-years old, we made a trip to Florida to visit Grammie, Grampie (Mom and Chuck) and Disneyworld and made many cherished memories. We stayed in the beautiful Contemporary Resort where the monorail runs through the building and the Characters' Café offered wonderful meal adventures for the little ones. This would be the most convenient location when we needed to go back for a rest, medications and a breathing treatment.

On the second day of our vacation I intentionally wore bright colors and told Josh that if for any reason he needed to find me, he should look for my vivid red shorts and brilliant yellow top. Later, I had changed my clothes for the evening before we went to the hotel's enormous game room

---

[28] . A bone age study helps doctors estimate the maturity of a child's skeletal system. It's usually done by taking a single X-ray of the left wrist, hand, and fingers. - KidsHealth

and remained near the door helping myself to some popcorn while Josh continued on with his dad to play one of the many games.

After a few minutes, Josh left his dad, saying he was going to find me. The huge game room was crowded. Josh, still looking for the bright color combination, walked right behind me and out the door. At about the same time, I found his dad and asked where Josh was. We both immediately panicked.

Although we had gone to Disney World some years after the Adam Walsh murder took place in Florida, that's the image that instantly exploded in my mind. The whole incident seemed like an hour long but in reality, was probably less than ten minutes in duration. We quickly searched the game room and then ran out toward the lobby where a blessed, wonderful clerk was leading Josh toward us. We thanked her profusely and went outside to sit on a fountain wall where I hugged and rocked him and cried in my relief. This incident might not have had such a happy ending if not for God watching over us that day.

The fantastic fireworks on the lake next to the Contemporary Resort that evening helped us to recover from the trauma of the "lost" incident, as did the next couple days of touring Disney World and Epcot Center. I so much enjoyed the wonderful music emanating from hidden speakers. Josh was especially fascinated by the fountains that would shoot out a short burst of water that swiftly disappeared somewhere undetectable. He also loved meeting Disney characters and experiencing the numerous attractions so well presented at the Resorts. Thank goodness for many of these attractions that we were able to ride, a welcome rest for Josh's overburdened lungs. We rode the monorail between "Kingdoms" that also provided some downtime.

Returning to Grammie and Grampie's winter Florida home, Josh was able to do some fishing, forever one of his favorite pastimes. It was, without question, a memorable trip and we had many pictures to help us reminisce.

That same year, the Buffalo Children's Hospital pediatric pulmonologist, Dr. Cropp, moved to New York City to teach at Columbia University. This resulted in the closing of the Buffalo Children's Hospital Outpatient Lung Clinic, a traumatic loss for us. Without a pulmonologist to routinely follow Josh, Dr. McConnell referred us to Children's Hospital of Pittsburgh (CHP) where he had trained.

The Pulmonology Clinic and its staff would soon come to be a very familiar second home. During our first visit at CHP, we met a very friendly pulmonologist, Dr. Blakeslee Noyes. It was always a joy to see his smiling face and we were treated with empathy and concern by the entire staff.

Our first CHP visit to the Pulmonology Clinic was in May 1989, and we were back again in August. Josh normally had a PFT on each of our Pittsburgh visits with a spattering of frequent EKGs and chest x-rays. Eye tests continued to be mandatory to check for development of cataracts due to his ongoing prednisone requirements. Very slowly he was gaining weight and growing in height, so next we were referred to a Nutritionist for recommendations on improving his caloric intake.

One day I noticed that the gum tissue was pulling away from Josh's lower front teeth, threatening to expose the roots, so I made an appointment with our local dentist. Yes, he had something called labial stripping and we were referred to the Dental Department at CHP in November of 1989 for confirmation and surgical repair.

During that appointment the initial novocaine administered was not successful, so the procedure was delayed until more could be administered. The additional local anesthesia was injected into two areas of a squirming little boy's mouth. The dentist was then able to remove a strip of tissue from the roof of Josh's mouth. He prepared the lower gums by scraping the surface area and grafted the tissue to his lower front gums. Shockingly, the dentist was not at all child-friendly, spoke gruffly to Josh for being uncooperative. He was obviously upset with the staff for inadequately administering the first local anesthetic, making Josh's experience so much more difficult, which deeply distressed me. The upside of this long, grueling ordeal was being able to pamper Josh by ordering his favorite, Chicken Alfredo, from Room Service at our hotel afterwards. Sore and tired, he was able to gingerly savor his delicious supper.

The next day we went to our appointment at the CHP Pediatric Chest Clinic. He had a routine chest x-ray as well as PFTs prior to the clinic visit. At this point the pulmonologists deemed his DIP was stable from a symptomatic point of view. His chest x-ray was unchanged from the one done in April of 1988. Thankfully, there were no changes in his therapeutic regimen this day.

I recall one trip - of many - to Pittsburgh, Jan had nearly run a red light and we immediately heard a siren. We looked around quickly and realized it was Josh in the back seat, sounding like a very authentic siren! We all had (a relieved) laugh about that.

In 1989 at age 8, Josh had a repeat Bone Age Study, showing his bone age to be nearly 4 years behind the chronologic age. His lung disease had unquestionably become the major factor in his lack of growth. He burned up the majority of his calories simply by struggling to breathe.

We were back in Pittsburgh in the end of January 1990 for a checkup and to have two teeth extracted. We saw them again in May when the plan was to wean Josh off Prednisone over a two-week period. The pulmonologists felt that his short stature and poor overall growth were likely due to his chronic lung disease as well as continued steroid use. The possibility of growth hormones was being considered, so we were scheduled for an Endocrine Department referral during our next appointment in August.

Mid-February 1991 saw us in the Department of Endocrinology for a re-evaluation of his growth stature. At that time, it was noted that during the previous November the prednisone dosage had been increased to 30 mg twice a day. It was then changed to 35 mg every other day and gradually decreased to 15 mg every other day. Growth hormone therapy was discussed and it was planned to have Josh admitted in the summer for intensive testing. Two lab tests, Insulin-like growth factor 1 (IGF-1) and Insulin-like growth factor-binding protein 3 (IGFBP-3) were drawn.

In September that same year, Josh was evaluated by the CHP Ophthalmology Services to rule out cataract formation by a slit lamp exam. Thank goodness, the results were entirely within normal limits.

Complaining of vague knee pain for several years, Josh, at age 10, had his knees x-rayed for possible Osgood-Schlatter Disease.[29] A common source of knee pain in growing adolescents is an inflammation of the slightly protruding area just below the knee joint where the tendon from the patella attaches to the tibia. It was noted that both his knee caps remained almost completely cartilage. Bony formation of the patella normally occurs by 6 years. The films, however, showed no evidence of Osgood-Schlatter Disease.

---

[29] . Osgood-Schlatter Disease (OSD) is far less frightful than its name. Though it's one of the most common causes of knee pain in adolescents, it's really not a disease, but an overuse injury. - KidsHealth

CHAPTER 7

The Elementary Years

Fishing and hunting were two of Josh's many favorite pastimes. He bagged his first buck on his 13th birthday, had his picture taken for the paper and received a free breakfast at a local restaurant. He played with neighborhood friends in the treehouse Jan had built for him, but he most enjoyed his motorcycle and our four-wheeler.

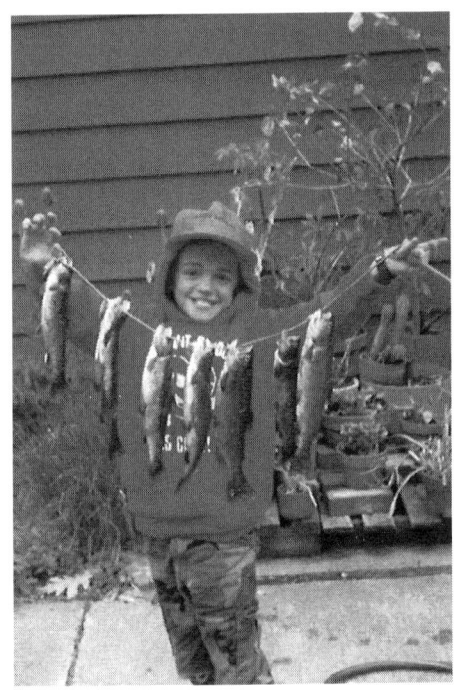

Happy fish!

Josh liked the water and tried swimming lessons at the "Y" at about age seven but his body fat was so low he literally was unable to stay afloat. He began junior bowling with classmates in the first grade and enjoyed it immensely, as it was something he could more easily compete in with schoolmates. We would go on weekends to practice with his 8-pound fluorescent bowling ball, sporting his name and etched with a dinosaur. He bowled into his early teens for as long as he was physically able.

I remember Josh telling me the story of a day when his class watched a movie in class in the second grade. Being so small for his age he could not see around the students in front of him. His friend Joey, very tall for his age, was at least a foot and a half taller and double in weight compared to Josh. Josh sat on his lap and was able to see as well as the rest of the class. They became good friends and loved to bowl and fish together.

It is rewarding to reflect upon all his accomplishments in spite of the challenges of his disease and continued health problems. After school one day, he shared a discussion they'd had in third grade about the use of condoms. Somewhat flabbergasted, I sat down in a rocker and he crawled up in my lap. I asked if he knew why they were used. He proceeded to explain, quite accurately, to my total surprise. What?! OK, that may be one explanation I might not need to clarify as much in the future.

Josh thoroughly enjoyed his Karate classes, making friends and practicing with the other students. Outside class, however, he found that his Karate training came in handy. One day when alone in the elementary school restroom, he was cornered by a bully and was forced to use his self-defense techniques. Needless to say, Josh was not harassed by this boy again. Office personnel caught wind of what had happened and covertly commended Josh for his handling of the situation. Apparently, the bully had struck before. Josh was truly a gentle soul, and continuously found it difficult to understand why people were so unkind, unfair and dishonest with each other.

Between Pittsburgh trips, we experienced many ER visits requiring x-rays, breathing treatments, EKGs, labs, scans, etc. Chest x-rays over time revealed chronic abnormalities, increasing hyperinflation and resultant pectus carinatum, as well as the post-surgical clips in his left upper chest from an open lung biopsy done at three months of age.[30, 31]

Results of Josh's Pulmonary Function Tests indicated obstructive and restrictive airways disease, only becoming worse and this thing called "lung transplant" was becoming more of a possibility as each year passed. It was now not so easy to dismiss.

While in karate, Josh became interested in dragons, a common symbol in Japanese mythology and folklore. He frequently drew dragons, feeling an affinity to the creature and sometimes wore a dragon ring or dragon pendant. Coincidentally, his high school mascot is a dragon. Because he passed away three years before graduating from high school, Josh will forever be my "incomplete dragon".

Just before his tenth birthday in November 1991, Josh was very ill with respiratory problems and was unable to go to school for two weeks. The hospital could do no more for him than what we were doing at home, so we were in a comfortable, warm, familiar place in the company of our beloved dogs. Rather than sitting at night by his bed in a rocker, I knew I'd get more rest lying down, so I moved him into our big bed and his dad slept in Josh's so I could continue to closely monitor his status. High fevers are so frightening, and I remember that at one point he was telling me about the Indians and horses he was seeing.

I gave him Tylenol and sponged him down frequently with a cool, wet cloth. Several times during the night I would administer breathing treatments and chest percussions. It was a grueling two weeks for us both, but gradually he felt better and was able to get up and around once again. It did take him quite a while to bounce back from that episode. One of his karate pictures was taken shortly after this episode and shows a beautiful smile but dark circles under his eyes in a gaunt face.

A few months following this illness we were required to provide medical records to the school because Josh had gone beyond the allowed sick days. The frequent and repeated illnesses took a great toll on his school attendance, schoolwork, his grades and eventually his self-esteem.

---

[30] . Hyperinflated lungs can be caused by obstructions in the passages that deliver air to your lung tissue. Air gets trapped within the lung and causes it to overinflate. Hyperinflation can also occur when the air sacs in your lungs become less elastic, which interferes with the expulsion of air from your lungs. - Mayo Clinic

[31] Pectus carinatum is an uncommon birth defect in which a child's breastbone protrudes outward abnormally. - Mayo Clinic

.

CHAPTER 8

Continuing Health Issues

At the end of July 1992, we were in the ER for wheezing, fever, and possible pneumonia. It was noted that his lung hyperinflation was increased, as well as the degree of pectus carinatum (barrel chest), and his heart was reported as slightly small. His ribs were giving way to the unrelenting expansion of his lungs. Again, in October he had a repeat "well chest x-ray" prior to our next Pittsburgh appointment that showed little change since the July study.

I tried to make light of many situations by having fun exchanges with Josh. I would tease him saying, "Josh, knock it off, you're acting like a kid!" His response then, and from that time on was, "Mom, I *am* a kid!" My reply was forever after was, with a double thumbs-up, "OK then, carry on!" I was so grateful that he was here, healthy enough and feeling well enough to act like a kid (Thank you, God!).

I recall the time the three of us had gone to a local restaurant. After the meal Jan pulled a bill from his wallet and teased Josh, "If you can tell me which president is on a fifty-dollar bill you can have it." Josh promptly responded, "Grant". In disbelief we all roared with laughter and the money was his.

Josh related the following anecdote repeatedly and with a great deal of glee. Josh and his dad had gone out to dinner together one evening, and the waitress took Josh's order. She then turned to his prematurely gray dad and said, "And what will your grandpa have?" They both cracked up and thoroughly enjoyed resharing this memory as it became a great joke between them.

April, 1993 found us back in Pittsburgh for a routine Pulmonology Clinic appointment. This visit found his height and weight to be below the

5th percentile. There was mention of coarse breath sounds in the lower lobes of both lungs, decreased breath sounds on the right and crackles were noted on both sides of the lungs.

During this visit, we learned that in a few months Dr. Noyes would be moving to St. Louis to work in a children's hospital there. This was another traumatizing loss to our family. We then met Dr. Geoffrey Kurland, one of the many pediatric pulmonologists at the Pulmonology Clinic. He immediately connected with Josh, relating his personal experience of lung disease, hospitalizations and his experience in the Martial Arts. Dr. Kurland quickly became Josh's (and our) favorite pulmonologist. I have a signed copy of his book, *My Own Medicine, A Doctor's Life as a Patient*.

Josh had an echocardiogram in mid-May, revealing a mitral valve prolapse with some other minor findings. Nothing needed to be done at that time, but it was to be routinely followed up.

CHAPTER 9

A Sad Split

The divorce. It was a no-brainer. Josh's dad and I had been discussing it for months. So as to not interfere with Josh's concentration in school, we opted to wait until the school year ended. The presentation of the concept to Josh, on the other hand, was a great deal more complicated and naturally rather emotional. What was best way to broach the subject without making him feel that he was in any way responsible? Our focus was on how to make him most comfortable with what was, from his perspective, a bad situation. Waiting until a Friday night after school was out for the year, we dove into this deep and difficult emotional pit. He cried and of course asked us, "Why?!!", somehow, as children will do, interpreting it to mean that this all was his fault. We assured him repeatedly that the decision had nothing to do with him, and that it would be better for us to be apart because his mom and dad just weren't treating each other all that well.

Josh had shared with me a couple of years before the story of a school friend and his sister who, after their parents' divorce, lived at one parent's home one week and the other the next. It seemed to me to be a distressing as well as a logistical nightmare, not to a mention total lack of stability, continuity, and peace in the children's lives. Josh had commented on how unhappy his friend was with this chaotic lifestyle. At all costs, I knew we had to make the transition as easy as possible for him to avoid mental and emotional challenges for this precious, already health-challenged child.

Looking for a home for Josh and me, I had decided that it should be fairly close to his dad's home to make visits much less complicated and also to be closer to the hospital. Fortunately, due to my management position at work, I was easily able to arrange a little time off to take Josh for his frequent routine lab tests, make sure he had breakfast, and then drive him to school.

It warmed my heart when several years later, after his death, my mom recounted that Josh had boasted to her a number of times that "I can see my dad whenever I want." I believe that is how our success was ultimately measured.

Arranging school meetings to clarify ongoing and anticipated health issues and recurring absences was no problem, and I was able to pick him up when he became ill at school. Fortune truly smiled down on me with my job and the freedom it afforded me. Even now, it is hard to imagine how the frequent medical tests, local physician office and Pittsburgh Pulmonary Clinic appointments would have worked so well had I not had this specific job. Bless my coworkers as they helped to make this possible. It's true; everything is as it is meant to be. Because of this flexibility, it worked best that Josh lived with me and visited his dad whenever possible. With Jan and a friend helping, we moved into our new home in July 1993.

Being close to his guy friends, Josh played street hockey with them as best he could. He was just grateful for living closer and being able to be with his friends more often. Happily, our home was five miles closer to town, but on the same road where his dad lived. Josh rode the same bus he had before with the same kids; the change was as seamless as possible. Simply a note from me would enable him to stay on the school bus longer and hop off at his dad's house.

We lived closer to Josh's friends, some within walking or biking distance but this eventually became a challenge for him. Merely walking half a block to the school bus stop left him short of breath. I would routinely give him a ride, especially in cold weather.

I have a memory of an amusing story Josh related to me of one of his friends (incidentally, a girl) defending him against a bully on the school bus. She had threatened the perpetrator with bodily harm if it ever happened again. He seemed to be proud to have such a friend to look out for him.

On the exceptionally snowy Halloween night of 1993, Mom had a heart attack, ended up in CCU and the next day was flown to St. Vincent's Hospital in Erie. While Chuck and I followed Mom to Erie, my wonderful new friend from work, Stacy, stayed with Josh and played pool, entertaining and getting to know each other. This was the beginning of my long and mutually supportive friendship with her. It was at this time that Stacy, knowing the back story, began calling him "Josh-Ua".

During our clinic visit on December 10, 1993, Josh's Pulmonary Function tests showed some alarming statistics. Among other findings, his total lung capacity was 179% of predicted and his residual volume 577% of predicted, indicating severe air trapping. When we briefly discussed the possibility of lung transplant, Josh became somewhat withdrawn and then wanted to leave the office. It was made clear that we were just talking about it, but it would not happen in the near future. We were to return in three to four months for re-evaluation.

By the time of our early May 1994 Clinic visit, Josh's PFT results were significantly worse than those of the previous December. The pulmonologist, Dr. Murphy, in his summary letter of this appointment to Dr. McConnell, stated that Josh had a high degree of functionality in the face of poor growth and decreasing lung function. Dr. Murphy surmised that this was probably related to Josh's positive attitude but also to some degree of misperception of the severity of his illness. Dr. Murphy felt that Josh may have been somewhat acclimatized to his degree of shortness of breath, but if his vital capacity (the maximum amount of air a person can expel from the lungs after a maximum inhalation) dropped any further, that then it would become quite noticeable.

CHAPTER 10

Challenges

The spring of 1994 brought bad news for Chuck, my kind and gentle stepfather. He was diagnosed with fast-growing Oat Cell Carcinoma of the lung. About 25 years earlier he had been treated with radiation therapy for throat cancer. Whether those were related or not, I have no idea, but this time at 85 years of age, he opted for no treatment. In August, Hospice was consulted and a hospital bed was delivered to their home. I was overwhelmed by what a wonderful, compassionate service these nurses provided. They made Chuck comfortable for his last weeks of life. What I learned about end-of-life then would haunt me for the next several years.

The story of the last weeks of Chuck's life is a sad, painful tale. Mom had suffered compression fractures of her lumbar spine and was confined to bed for several weeks. I suspect her injury occurred while helping to lift, turn and move Chuck in his bed.

On the second of August, we had a follow-up appointment at the CHP Pulmonology Clinic. Josh, at age 12, had actually lost weight since our prior appointment and weighed the same as he had 15 months before. His PFTs were changed very little, and Dr. Murphy's letter stated that Josh's entire health picture reflected a terrific degree of obstruction within the lungs. Again, when we spoke of transplant, Josh immediately became very quiet and withdrawn. He was clearly not ready to think about that and admitted that hearing it made him worry about dying. Dr. Murphy's real concern, stated in his summary letter, was that we may well run out of time for Josh regarding lung function and viability since the wait for his new lungs may well be over a year. Nevertheless, he was clearly not ready to take on that issue. The doctor further noted that no one *has* to undergo a lung transplantation and if Josh does not desire to do so, that was certainly within his rights. A transplant may not be an option Josh wanted. The writing was on the wall. Time was quickly running out for Josh.

His low weight was becoming a critical issue, and it was strongly recommended that we push calories and consider other ways to force him to at least parallel his growth curve pattern. We were told that as an alternative to an intake of adequate calories for growth, an NG tube would have to be considered, to prove or disprove how much of his failure to grow was caloric malnutrition. This was getting serious.

I am hard pressed to think of anything more excruciating and terrifying to a parent than seeing your child face his life-threatening health issues and being acutely aware that he is very likely looking at his own death. It is chilling, even now, reflecting on what Josh was going through at that time.

As Josh and I were returning from this appointment in Pittsburgh, we stopped at Mom and Chuck's house to visit on our way home. Sadly, we learned that he had passed away in the middle of the night. Mom knew that we would be traveling that day and deliberately hadn't called us with the heartbreaking news.

Sitting by Mom's bed, I consoled her, then shared the additional bad news: Josh was in end-stage (the last phase in the course of a progressive disease) pulmonary disease and now it was imperative that he be placed on the Transplant List. The burning question was: would he agree to this critical, life-saving surgery?

What a concept that was for me to absorb. *End-stage*. The mere mention of this phrase literally jarred my heart. The *end* of my child's life. OK God, let's kick this into high gear. Now what do I need to do to keep my child healthy and alive? This was an especially difficult time with numerous stressors; it was truly tough to remain rational and clear-headed.

When the day of Chuck's funeral arrived, Mom was still in so much pain she was unable to attend and although there was nothing else that could be done, she was unable to forgive herself. Stacy, such a good and now long-time friend, attended the funeral with me and was again so very supportive.

One month later, on September 6, we were back in the Pulmonology Clinic. By this time Josh, a black belt, had decided to give up participating in karate, representing a marked deterioration in his exercise tolerance. He was having difficulty with strenuous activities, for example, feeling out of breath after ascending a flight of stairs. For about three weeks he had been experiencing headaches which were waking him up in the middle of the night. Those were resolved by increasing his nighttime oxygen from 1 liter to 1½ liters.

According to Dr. Murphy, the increase in Josh's nighttime oxygen requirement represented the consequences of hypoxia due to severely reduced lung function.[32] Josh had only gained just over one pound in weight since August 2, and his height was unchanged. It was noted that while sitting quietly, he was having mild retractions and appeared pale. Initially, when the issue of transplant was again raised, Josh became quiet. However, he and I had been discussing this over the past month, becoming familiar with and perhaps more accepting of the concept. I also think that his recognition of his own decline played a large role in this. Stoicism was no longer able to carry him through the rough times. Those tough times had gradually morphed into tremendously horrible ones without him noticing; or rather, without his acknowledging them. It was no longer possible to avoid the inescapable truth. The "Big T" was looming...without it, there was only one remaining outcome.

The other major concern continued to be Josh's failure to grow and gain weight. Josh was trying very hard to maintain a goal of 2,000 calories a day and showed just a small amount of weight gain. His goal as of this appointment was increased to 2,300 calories daily. Josh knew in order to dodge the NG tube "bullet", this was a very important goal to try to attain. The possibility of a G-tube was also discussed at this time. A G-Tube, or gastrostomy tube is inserted into the stomach through the abdomen, delivering nutrition directly to the stomach.[33]

Dr. Murphy's general impression at this appointment was that Josh continued to demonstrate slow but steady deterioration. There were a few changes made in his medical therapy and a change of his antibiotic. Arrangements were made for the homecare company who provided

---

[32] . A lower-than-normal concentration of oxygen in arterial blood, as opposed to anoxia, a complete lack of blood oxygen. Hypoxia will occur with any interruption of normal respiration. - MedicineNet

[33] . A gastrostomy tube (also called a G-tube) is a tube inserted through the abdomen that delivers nutrition directly to the stomach. It's one of the ways doctors can make sure kids with trouble eating get the fluid and calories they need to grow. - KidsHealth

his oxygen concentrator to begin monitoring Josh's nighttime oxygen saturations (oximetry).[34]

Josh's name was given to Tammy, our Transplant Coordinator, who would, per my request, try to put us in contact with other families of lung transplant recipients. Another appointment was made for next month. Many lab tests would be done at that visit, as suggested by the transplant team. An appointment would also be made for us to meet with a surgeon.

On October 13, we had another appointment to re-evaluate Josh's growth. Happily, his weight showed a modest improvement over the previous month, heading towards, rather than away from the 5th percentile. He was making a valiant effort to gain weight; he did gain in height, but, oh so very little.

---

[34] . The measuring of oxygen saturation of the blood by means of an oximeter. – Dictionary.com

CHAPTER 11

Transplant Evaluation

In early November 1994, just two weeks prior to his 13th birthday, Josh was admitted to Children's Hospital of Pittsburgh November 13th-16th for the pre-transplant evaluation. We met with a Pain Management Physician, Pulmonologists, Dietician and a Psychologist. He had the following tests: Pulmonary Function Testing, Pulmonary Exercise text, chest x-ray, Echocardiogram, MUGA Scan (multigated acquisition scan, a nuclear medicine test designed to evaluate the function of the right and left ventricles of the heart), multiple Lab tests, Chest CT Scan, Abdominal Ultrasound.

The psychological and social evaluation took place privately; the psychologist interviewed Jan and me and then spoke to Josh alone. With amusement, I clearly remember Josh's comments to us when the psychologist's interview with him had been completed. We returned to his room and asked how it had gone. It appeared that he had been rather offended because he informed us that when she had asked if he knew where he was, he pointed to a sign on the wall across from his bed and with assurance responded, "It says Children's Hospital of Pittsburgh right there!" I believe he passed *that* test with flying colors!

Josh was placed in the UNOS (United Network for Organ Sharing) Network. UNOS had developed an online database system to collect, store, analyze and publish all Organ Procurement Transplant Network (OPTN) data pertaining to the patient waiting list, organ matching, and transplants performed. This system contains data regarding every organ donation and transplant event occurring in the United States since October 1, 1987. Transplant professionals use it to register transplant candidates on the national waiting list, match them with donated organs, and enter vital medical data on candidates, donors and transplant recipients.

Josh's case was discussed at the Cardiopulmonary Transplant Conference on November 21, 1994 and his name was placed on the UNOS registry waiting list the same day.

During our next appointment on December 15, we met with Dr. Bartley Griffith, the transplant surgeon. He was quite frank with us and discussed in general terms how the surgery would be done, describing the "clamshell" technique that would be used.

This visit also reflected a moderate weight gain, but unchanged height, both still well below the 5th percentile. Now on 20 mg daily prednisone and 2 liters of oxygen, Josh had started to wake up in the middle of the night needing a breathing treatment. Because of these nocturnal symptoms we began using Serevent rather than Albuterol to take advantage of the longer-lasting benefits. The pulmonologist stated in his letter to Dr. McConnell regarding this visit that if the symptoms persist, a gastroesophageal reflux workup should be considered.

Our next appointment on January 24, 1995 it was noted that Josh was again experiencing a marked decrease in exercise tolerance. Classes at school were arranged so that he would not need to climb stairs. Josh had missed a considerable amount of school due to his shortness of breath and wheezing. This month he showed weight loss, appeared pale, and was in mild distress. It was also noted that his breath sounds in the lower lobes of the lungs were markedly decreased at this time, which was an alarming finding.

Josh was again experiencing nighttime headaches, a sign of hypoxia. Oximetry would determine the percentage of oxyhemoglobin in his blood and indicate whether his oxygen requirements would need to be increased. The oximetry was performed over a three-day period, results showing that his lowest oxygen saturation was in the low 80s. These findings indicated that Josh's nighttime oxygen therapy dose would have to be increased. Our pulmonary clinic appointments continued on a monthly basis with no improvements noted.

At that time, we were put in contact with Make-A-Wish, a wonderful organization granting the wishes of children with life-threatening medical conditions. A local volunteer representative visited our home and asked Josh what his wish might be. He asked if he could meet Dale Earnhardt and see a NASCAR race. His health unfortunately was not sufficient to withstand such an adventure at that time. It would have to wait until after transplant...if we could hold on that long.

CHAPTER 12

Preparing for Transplant

Shortly before Josh's transplant evaluation we had learned about "Caring for Life", a non-profit group that assisted the families of Warren County children with life-threatening illnesses. This support group was established by the administrator, Linda Sivak. Linda worked tirelessly arranging fund-raising events such as spaghetti and pancake suppers, gun raffles, donation cans and many others, giving 100% of the proceeds toward families of many critically ill children in Warren County, Pennsylvania.

Through Caring for Life, resources were provided for fuel, toll fees, parking, meals, housing at Ronald McDonald House, etc. for our frequent CHP appointment trips. Shortly after the transplant evaluation, an article appeared in the local newspaper describing Josh's chronic disease, the deterioration of his health and impending double-lung transplant. The article also announced the first of many fundraisers organized by "Caring for Life". Post-transplant, Linda had arranged a wonderful paddle-boat ride on Lake Erie and a lunch afterwards for all her "kids" and parents. There were even TV cameras documenting the outing and an interview with Josh.

With a full heart, I would like to thank Linda for the wonderful memories, her generosity of time, funds, love for all her precious clients, providing support for them and their anxious families, as well as for the significant part she played in our life story. I will always be indebted to her and admire her selflessness, generosity of love, time and funding.

Through an appointment with a CHP Social Work representative and as part of the transplant evaluation, we were informed about our eligibility to use Ronald McDonald House. This would be so much less expensive than the hotel we had been utilizing when we were required to stay overnight for early next-morning medical tests, procedures and Pulmonology Clinic appointments.

The house we utilized was a beautiful old Victorian home, four stories and fairly close to the hospital. There were multiple comfortable living rooms, kitchens, bedrooms, shared bathrooms as well as TV and game rooms. The kitchens were stocked with essentials such as milk, juice, bread, etc. It was an amazing place to rest and relax. We retrieved sheets for our beds upon arrival and removed them at the end of our stay and washed and dried them in the provided laundry room.

During one such visit, we met a family from the Carolinas whose teenage son had handled a dried sea urchin at school. Tragically, this resulted in liver failure due to the poison he had absorbed. They were living at Ronald Mc Donald House, awaiting a liver donor. I sometimes wonder what the outcome was for this family. I pray they did have a donor in time.

Soon after his evaluation, when Josh was placed on the Transplant List, we received a beeper to keep us constantly in touch with Tammy, our Transplant Coordinator. Unfortunately, there were no cell phones at that time. Sure enough, on a dark and rainy night in April 1995, 'the call' came. I'm sure my heart rate and blood pressure were sky-high during that trip. We hustled down to CHP where Josh had his labwork done, had an IV placed, was on a stretcher and ready to go into the operating room. It was at this point where we were told that preliminary testing of the donor lungs revealed that the patient had aspirated vomit. These lungs were not viable. The surgery was off. What a incredible disappointment this was, especially in light of Josh's continuing deteriorating health status. Starting out the trip on an adrenalin high, we had hit rock bottom late that night, traveling back home, quite saddened. Frankly, I was depressed, knowing this was to be perhaps his only opportunity for the life-saving procedure. We had been psyched and ready to do this.

By mid-May 1995, Josh could no longer attend school due to the rapid progression of his disease which was causing severe shortness of breath resulting in profound weakness and fatigue. The doctors had called it "end-stage disease", a term that sent chills straight to my heart. The thought, "Would a donor come in time?" was constantly on my mind. Repeated and frequent prayers were going out. Hang on, Josh, hang on!

One morning I had fabricated a story for Josh, that we had to go to school to obtain books so he could work with his tutor. We needed to enter by way of the gym and gathered there was his entire class and teachers. Josh was presented with a check from donations, extra lunch money and spare change that was collected in a large jar throughout the year. He was so surprised, looking quite self-conscious from all the attention but grinning the whole time. The love and generosity of these children and teachers were overwhelming for us both. Josh was privileged to have known them; I only hope they felt the same way.

With my friend Bea's urging, we visited her brother Randy who had received a liver transplant, and his wife Ann. We were readily welcomed into their home to discuss Randy's transplant. They shared stories that related to all aspects of the transplant process. Randy offered to show Josh what he referred to as his "shark bite" scar, but Josh declined, trying to take in all the information, already having enough to digest.

Knowing only that his donor came from Louisiana, Randy joked that he now had a craving for Cajun food. In retrospect, I recognized that I had forced Josh to face this head-on. But I felt that if he met someone who had already gone through and survived an organ transplant, he would feel less anxious with his own impending surgery. As a result, Ann and Randy became dear friends and staunch supporters for Josh and myself and later my local transplant support group, Close to the Heart.

I might add that, remarkably, some transplant recipients have an interesting perspective on this subject, which demonstrates that this could be a very real possibility. Their experience is credited to something called Cellular Memory Theory or Cell Memory Phenomenon. The scientific world does not agree on the fact of its existence. However, many organ recipients may argue the point.[35] I'd like to believe it's true, yet another gift from the donor.

After recent research and reading a book about just that, I have learned that this phenomenon is known as "cell memory". This seems to be a variation of body memory, the yet to be proven scientifically hypothesis that memories can be stored in individual cells.

In addition, I took Josh to a local psychologist, ostensibly to better prepare him mentally for the stressful process. In retrospect, I have to wonder whether this was more for myself than it was for him. God Bless him for tolerating all my "pre-transplant prep baloney". Without saying it in so many words, he seemed to have the attitude, "Let's get this over with

---

[35] . http://timcusack.com/tag/cellular-memory/

so I can get on with my life." Hey, I understood that he had more important things to do; it must be a guy thing.

On July 12, 1995, we arrived at Three Rivers Stadium in Pittsburgh, PA, for Josh to watch a pre-game practice, and then the game, where he met and procured autographs from the manager, Jim Leland and player, Mark P. Johnson as well as others.

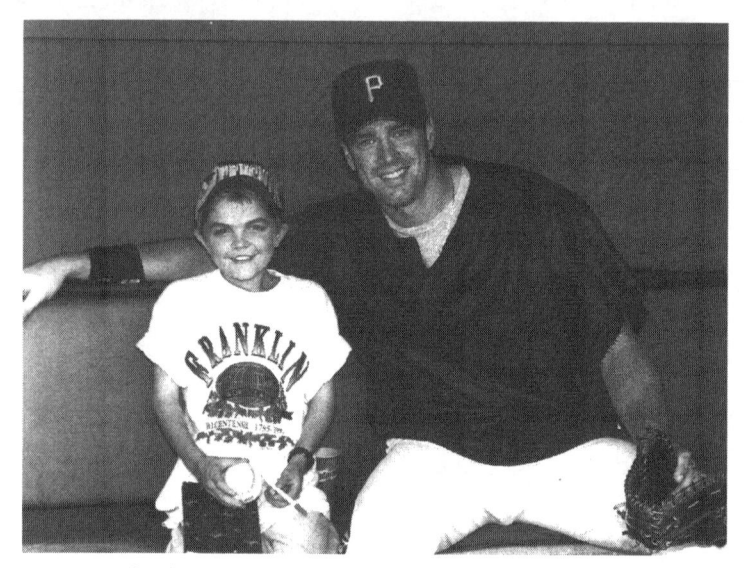

In the dugout! Josh (age 13) and Mark P. Johnson (First Baseman for the Pittsburgh Pirates) together at Three Rivers Stadium in July, 1995, just one week before transplant.

CHAPTER 13

The Call

On July 19, 1995, at work and in a hospital manager's meeting, I received a phone call from our Transplant Coordinator, asking how long it would take us to get to Pittsburgh. When I looked at the room full of managers and answered, "We can be there in 3 hours," everyone in the room stood, cheered and applauded, fully aware of the significance of this statement. To this day, I remember and appreciate the support I received from so many friends and coworkers.

Reflecting on that day, it seems really insane to ask someone to drive a loved one 150 miles while remaining calm and rational. After "the call", calm and rational feelings were nowhere near what I was experiencing. And so naturally, despite my constant efforts to keep the gas tank full for the past seven months for what I knew (or more accurately, *prayed*) would be that inevitable call, my gas tank was down to half, not quite enough to get that off my pre-transplant to-do list.

I stopped at a local full-service gas station to fill up but didn't/couldn't wait for the attendant to come to the car. I put the gas cap on the roof of the Blazer and filled the tank myself. I'm pretty sure I paid, because I must have been doing a tortured dance in my agonizing need to get the heck out of there as quickly as possible. When I picked Josh up at Mom's home in Pittsfield, I realized that the fuel door cover was still open, the gas cap no longer on the roof, but apparently bouncing along the road somewhere behind me.

My heart must have been pounding audibly and I was focused only on getting to the 'Burgh quickly and safely. Thinking back, I imagine that this stress, along with the limiting time factor inherent in recovered organs, is probably the basis of changing the transport of patients to the hospital by helicopter. However, family still have the long difficult road trip ahead of them with any number of wild thoughts coursing through their brains. For me, there's little memory of this trip, I just know that Josh and I anxiously gripped each other's hand and spoke very little. This was really going to happen! My precious son was about to receive a second chance at life.

It was 4 p.m. when we finally arrived at the hospital (the three-hour trip made in record two-and-a-half hours), and Josh was whisked away for insertion of IVs, last minute lab testing, etc. It was a whirlwind of nurses and doctors rushing here and there, readying equipment and organizing details, performing their jobs. When they took him away, my anxiety increased by a factor of probably 1000. Heart pounding, I looked around to see if Jan had arrived yet. Yes, I had been rational enough to remember to call him. I needed someone sane to hold onto, emotionally as well as physically. Josh was taken into the OR at 4:30 p.m., a set of new lungs awaiting. Josh's small stature required size—not age—appropriate lungs, and hers would certainly go to good use. I sometimes wonder how many other recipients' lives this precious little girl saved and enhanced.

I made phone calls to family and friends, blindly stared at the TV and at others in the waiting room, wringing my hands, wondering what their individual stories were and if they could possibly be as distressed as I was. There were all kinds of terrified, disorganized thoughts flitting through my head; things that could not be said aloud. I was imagining the clamshell surgery, as described months ago by the surgeon. I guess I should have appreciated the fact that I was undeniably not in my right mind during this extraordinarily stressful period.

Truly agonizing, our time in the Surgical Waiting Room dragged on hour after hour. Jan and I had been told that during his surgery, Josh would be placed on a Cardiopulmonary Bypass Machine (CBM).[36] This was but one of many devastatingly painful visuals I experienced that night in the waiting room. It was impossible to shut the mind off, adrenalin seemingly coursing through the body at the speed of light. Total exhaustion would eventually follow, but not for days into the future. I think we had an adrenalin overload for quite a while.

---

[36] . A cardiopulmonary bypass machine (CBM) is commonly known as a heart-lung bypass machine. It is a device that does the work of providing blood (and oxygen) to the body when the heart is stopped for a surgical procedure. - verywellhealth

It was close to midnight before one of the surgeons came out to give us an update. The surgery was almost completed. The lungs and their vessels had been attached; now another team was "closing" (suturing and stapling) his little chest back up. What horrible, racing images this implanted in my brain; it was impossible to control the emotions. Through the haze, we received the information that Josh would be moved to the Recovery Room and later to ICU; we could see him—although only briefly—in a couple hours. At the moment he was holding his own, the best we could hope for right now. He had survived the transplant and fortified by this optimistic report, we waited impatiently for several more hours; I was praying more intensely than I ever had before.

When we were finally permitted into the ICU isolation room to see him, Josh was sedated, unconscious and on a ventilator, which was doing the breathing for him. At 13 years old and just over 50 pounds, he looked so small, pale, delicate and vulnerable. I cried, feeling helpless, yet so very grateful he was alive. Thank You, God, Thank You God, Thank You God!

I observed a collection of IV tubings running from bags and an assortment of measurement devices. An IV had been inserted into a vein on the right side of Josh's neck, a ventilator tube through his mouth into his trachea. There was also a catheter in his bladder, a total of four chest tubes, two on each side of his lower chest, and more staples from one armpit to the other than I'd ever seen. Days later we counted the staples together and came up with 80. My heart pounded with unimaginable anxiety. I pushed his hair back, gently held his hand, cried and thanked God my little boy was not awake; the pain would have been unbearable for us both. He needed a couple days on the ventilator to start the healing process.

Gradually over the next three days, Josh was weaned off the ventilator. Then he was moved out of the ICU isolation room and moved to the general ICU ward, a frightening yet promising step on the long and complicated path to recovery. I recall with great trepidation the next early morning visit when I could see that he was clearly in extreme distress.

Josh leaned on his elbows on the bedside table with a look of panic on his face, he asked me, "Mom, am I going to die?" I thought I'd drop dead on the floor right then and there. His imploring look and heart-wrenching question are burned into my brain for all time. I see this scene in my mind now as if it had just happened yesterday. Eerily, it was not to be the last time I would see that terrified look in his eyes.

Alarmed and with a pounding heart, I immediately called out to a nurse and requested pain medication for him *STAT*. What I actually meant was *yesterday!* I was to learn that Pain Management is not an exact science. Each patient responds to drugs differently and sometimes an alternate pain medication would be necessary. Josh needed to learn to ask for his Percocet well before the pain became unbearable. Lesson learned.

Finally, after several days, Josh was moved to a private room. This quickly came to feel very comfortable and was like home to us. It was wonderful to be alone together in a quieter, less frenzied environment where we could talk and reflect on what was and would be happening. There was a chair available that converted into a cot, and a shower in his room, so I didn't even need to leave except to eat. Many times, I didn't even want to do that. I was hypervigilant for weeks on end. It's surprising my adrenals didn't burn out.

In a very short time, the walls were plastered with hundreds of notes, cards, pictures, posters and quantities of other memorabilia. Josh received a certificate from Rick Johnson's Shotokan Karate Academy, stating that he was now an honorary second-degree Black Belt, something he was ever so proud of. This certificate was prominently displayed on the wall among all his cards.

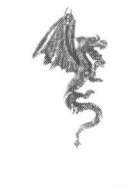

CHAPTER 14

Post-Transplant Challenges

We soon learned that Josh had developed Cytomegalovirus (CMV), originating with his donor, not a rare occurrence.[37] Sources of CMV infections in transplant recipients could include latent reactivation, donor-transmitted virus, and virus present in donor white blood cells. Well, there's another medication added to the list. Simple enough; thank you, God.

Hearing helicopters continually landing and taking off right above Josh's room caused a bit of distraction until we became accustomed to the racket. I slept and showered in his room and tended to many of Josh's needs. In the early days following transplant, we valiantly fought boredom by playing cards and other games provided by the hospital. We would admire the plastering of his walls with cards, notes and letters and discussed many of the medical issues that arose. Together, we requested a pass for a short trip out-of-house when that eventually became an option. I encouraged and supported him and helped him to schedule selected video games and equipment for delivery to his room. What an immense thrill and clear step in a positive direction to be able to escape the increasingly confining hospital environment for a short time! I felt very fortunate that I was allowed to stay so close, keeping watch over him, monitoring how he was feeling. In retrospect, I'm sure that I also drove him bonkers, just one of my many responsibilities as a mom. I hovered. I watched. I worried. I advocated.

---

[37] . CMV is a member of the herpes virus group, which also includes herpes simplex virus, varicella-zoster virus (which causes chickenpox) and Epstein-Barr virus (which causes infectious mononucleosis). These viruses share a characteristic ability to remain dormant within the body over a long period. – MedicineNet

One morning a week after surgery, I noticed while helping Josh to turn in bed that his lower back around the sacrum was becoming quite red. He had been positioned on his back for days. I noticed the skin was beginning to break down and would develop into a bed sore unless we took immediate measures. I promptly called a nurse and requested an "egg-crate" mattress for him, and started turning him ever so slightly, propping him slightly with a rolled towel to prevent the constant pressure on the same location on his back.

Initially the Pain Management team reminded Josh that he had to alert the nurse early before his pain became too severe, otherwise it would be slow to get back under control. Always stoic, he had never endured this unexpected pain intensity, so in the very beginning he had difficulty learning to ask for his Percocet on a timely basis. However, he soon learned to recognize the increasing pain and to request the meds appropriately. OK, one challenge defeated, so many more in store.

Josh was thrilled when he learned he was permitted to reserve video games and movies for his room. The more he had to entertain himself the better, as he was tethered by multiple chest tubes and IV lines inside a room for an undetermined amount of time. Gradually things improved. First one tube from each side of his chest was removed and, in a few days—and a few chest x-rays later—the other two chest tubes were eliminated.

Where the chest tubes had been removed, his skin had been pinched together and stapled to assist in wound closure. Josh was hunched over so as not to pull on the tender area around the staples. To me this looked very painful and when I closely examined the area a day later, I was able to see why. The staples were actually tearing through the skin when he tried to stand upright. I prayed that this phase would soon be complete. I found myself frequently wishing it could be me experiencing this instead of him. Again, this was not the last time I made this appeal.

After what seemed like an eternity, at last all the chest tubes were removed; we felt so liberated! First, I took him in a wheelchair with his IVs around the floor and visited a game room where there were presentations by volunteers and nurses. It was both an exciting and nervous time for both of us to get out and see new faces and places.

One of our first outings was across and down the hall to the "tub room", where Josh had his first real bath since his surgery. We were both tentative, and I gently washed around his tender surgical areas. It was a new but stressful and exhausting experience, then back to bed for a rest!

We had company one weekend, and they seemed to be having trouble with their camera. Josh asked to see it so he could check it out. Rotating it to take a look, he accidentally took an exposure and it flashed intensely in his face. Everyone cracked up, including Josh, though his laughter caused a lot of pain to his recently traumatized body. He unsuccessfully attempted to suppress his laughter, making the incident even more hilarious. The poor guy, we were having a huge laugh, and perhaps a bit of tension release, at his expense!

In a few more days some of the staples across his chest began to be removed and replaced with Steri Strips. Again, wishing it could have been me instead. To add to the torment there were daily needle sticks for various labs. Some of the nurses and lab techs were willing to take blood from his IV; others would refuse and used a vein instead. You would think after all he'd been through, he wouldn't mind the venous sticks anymore, but the whole experience seemed to do the reverse, and sensitize him even more to needles. It was all he could do to cooperate fully with the tech doing the lab draws.

I remember the day he first went to Physiotherapy. The therapists had him walking, although slowly, up and down a series of about seven steps, a real challenge so soon after his surgery. We were just trying to build his strength back up after a couple weeks in bed.

One night after 11 p.m. the corridor floor outside Josh's room was being stripped and the toxic odor was seeping into the room. I was quite annoyed that Josh was exposed to not only the noise, but worse, the noxious odor. I immediately informed the night nurses how I felt about this incident. I laid down blankets at the bottom of the door in an attempt to block the fumes.

There were frequent treatments to help clear the lungs of mucus, an automated machine being used for chest percussion. This was obviously a very uncomfortable procedure initially for Josh due to the painful areas where his chest was opened to insert and attach the lungs and blood vessels.

Soon Josh received a Broviac catheter, inserted into his upper chest, under anesthesia.[38] This is a soft IV catheter inserted to avoid the need for repeated peripheral IV sticks. It is placed directly into a central vein, usually in the neck, upper chest or groin. The catheter is then fed into a position just above the heart. In general, the catheter is tunneled under the skin and

---

[38] . A Broviac®/Hickman® central venous line (CVL) is a special intravenous (IV) line inserted under the skin on the chest wall and into a large vein that leads to the heart. It's used in children and teens who need IV therapy for a long time. CVLs are helpful for: Chemotherapy and other medications. - CHEO

brought out on the chest or thigh away from the site where it enters the vein, theoretically preventing bacteria from gaining access to the catheter.

A sterile dressing was placed over the area where the Broviac catheter exited his chest, an important barrier to prevent infection. An additional Steri Strip dressing was placed on his chest where the catheter entered the vein to help hold it in place. Because Josh would be discharged with the catheter in place, I was taught how to change this dressing, a nerve-wracking process at first. I also learned to flush the catheter with saline in order to keep it clear. Several times we were required to go to the hospital to have it flushed with Urokinase to dissolve the clot which had formed over the catheter opening, blocking it off.

These things had to be constantly checked, adjusted and balanced. My role, I felt, was to be Josh's advocate and I was grateful to have the job. But sometimes I did such a good job that at least in my own eyes, I truly must have driven him up the wall and to be honest sometimes vice-versa.

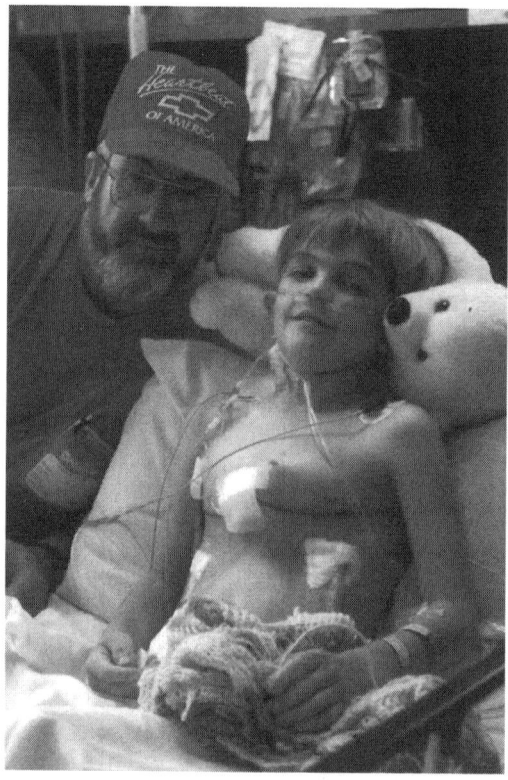

Jan, Josh and Klondike

All Josh's medications were critical and life-saving, but they do have some negative side effects, including cataracts and diabetic complications due to high doses of steroids given. Special anti-rejection medications—immunosuppressants—are used to suppress the organ recipient's immune system, preventing rejection of the donated organ.[39] Initially daily lab testing is required to assure correct dosing and to detect the presence of viruses, potentially deadly to the patient. Regular lung biopsies, done at CHP, also became a part of Josh's routine post-transplant care.

We had to slog through the day-to-day trials of depression and guilt ("Someone died so I can live"), a common post-transplant emotion. I was learning the names, doses, timing and use of endless strange medications. There were secondary infections and viruses due to the immunity suppression; then there were additional medications to treat and prevent further complications. We survived daily relying on each other's strength and love as well as additional support of compassionate family and friends.

Thrush (oral candidiasis), a fungal infection, raised its ugly head and Josh was started on a permanent Nystatin "swish" regimen to keep it controlled. Thrush risk factors include use of antibiotics and corticosteroids, both of which Josh was prescribed post-transplant. A CHP dentist examined Josh a couple of weeks' post-transplant and explained to us how important it was to keep his mouth clean, infection continually a concern for any organ transplant recipient.

Shortly after transplant, I speculated whether additional intense emotional support should have been provided for recipient and family. Our Transplant Coordinator did her best to help us in this area, but I must say, the three to four weeks following transplant was an extremely emotionally difficult time for both Josh and me. I was stressed from the start, aware that transplant is not a cure, but should be considered simply as a different set of health challenges. Reflecting on this, I now realize the team's primary responsibility was for the physical pieces of the organ transplant puzzle, but nevertheless, what an enormously emotional roller coaster this experience evolved into.

---

[39] . An agent that can suppress or prevent the immune response. Immunosuppressants are used to prevent rejection of a transplanted organ and to treat autoimmune diseases such as psoriasis, rheumatoid arthritis, and Crohn's disease. - MedicineNet

CHAPTER 15

Post-Transplant Recuperation

During the transplant admission, it was always a wonderful boost for both of us to have Josh's (and my) favorite pulmonologist, Dr. Kurland, stop by. We couldn't see him enough; he was an old, comfortable friend, a wonderful familiar face. Always positive, teasing and joking with Josh, Dr. K. helped significantly to brighten his spirits and outlook.

Several times I spoke with our transplant coordinator, in tears, stressed to the max, discussing Josh and how cantankerous and uncooperative he had been with me. She was sympathetic, patiently explaining that Josh's moodiness was most certainly a combination of being so soon post major surgery, numerous new medications, burgeoning hormones, constant pain and the isolation he was required to endure. Maybe all that plus my sky-high levels of adrenaline had negative effects on him and me. OK, together we can get through this.

Yes, he was in the hospital away from family, friends and Cinnamon (his docile red and white Basset Hound). Anyone would be a little crazy under these circumstances. So, when a Basset therapy dog was offered, we agreed immediately and looked forward to her visit. Contrary to my expectations, a picture of Josh with his hand on her back clearly shows how miserable he was being away from home and how much he missed his sweet buddy, Cinnamon.

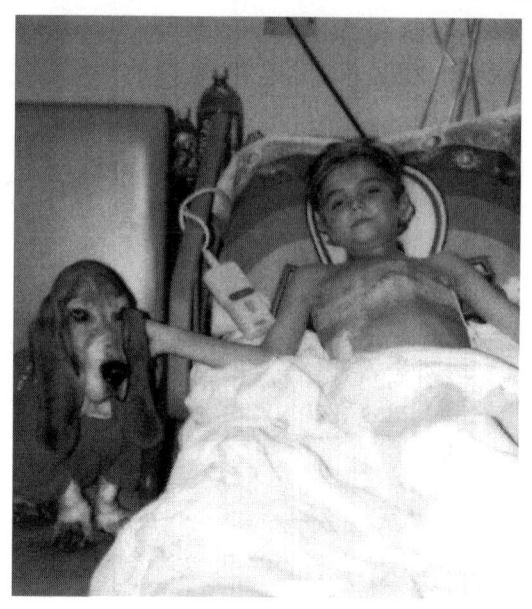

Josh and Therapy Dog

    One afternoon in early August, Josh put on a loose t-shirt and a pair of shorts, free at last from the restrictive chest tubes. I put him in a wheelchair and took the elevator down to the cafeteria. What an adventure and how wonderful it felt to be able to plan the "escape". After two isolated weeks, getting out of that room was almost as good as going to Disney World! On the elevator, we encountered a very young girl with an IV being pushed by her mother. Josh didn't say anything at the time but asked after they had exited why the child had no hair. I explained that it appeared the child had cancer and was perhaps being treated by chemotherapy. He ruminated on that for quite a while and, I believe, saw how fortunate he truly was.

    On our increasingly frequent outings, Josh would ask to make a side trip to the gift shop where there were books, games, puzzles and other kinds of entertainment. This was a great distraction and provided hours of enjoyment.

    There was a great restaurant within walking distance of the hospital which we had previously visited in conjunction with our Lung Clinic visits. With permission and a pass, we took a scary wheelchair trip down a steep hill for a very enjoyable lunch. Josh was so thankful to finally be able to escape the confines of his room and the hospital. The restaurant was across the street from a scrubs shop where later I was able to find some interesting wear for work. Several times we went to the UPMC cafeteria for a meal, which was offering more interesting fare and definitely different surroundings than the CHP cafeteria.

On another day-pass, we had great get-away trip to the Carnegie Science Center. We did a quick tour and took time for lunch while we were there. Josh tired quickly, but we were both grateful we were able to obtain passes. These short trips provided a welcomed interruption to the monotony we found within our four white walls. In addition, I had to feel thankful that he felt well enough to partake in these outings, which signified that he was well on his way to recovery.

In mid-August, about three weeks after transplant, one of the frequent chest x-rays revealed a pneumonia, resulting in a course of antibiotics being given. Later, when I went home for a short two-day break, Jan came to the 'Burgh and took Josh on a pass to Hooters for lunch. I was shocked when I learned of this trip, but it was a once-in-a-lifetime experience and a fun trip for Josh. The girls fussed over him and he returned with a keepsake shirt covered with the signatures of many of the staff. Josh was grinning! OK, no harm done. Undeniably, this was an unconventional yet exciting distraction from a 13-year-old boy's daily hospital routine.

After his post-transplant hospital discharge, we went to our wonderfully familiar and comfortable Ronald McDonald House for a few days. This provided practice at being in the home environment with the added confidence that help was nearby if needed. When we were allowed to actually go home, it was very daunting, yet it gave us an exhilarating sense of freedom. We now had a whole new normal.

Following Josh's transplant, we were back in Pittsburgh in a few weeks for a follow-up visit and testing and learned that a family, traveling from a different culture, was also lodging at Ronald McDonald House. The alert and considerate house manager informed us we weren't going to be able to stay in our regular room. Due to their customs, this family stood at, rather than sat on the toilet. Because Josh was immunosuppressed, he knew that Josh could not be exposed to probable contamination. Appreciatively, we took a room on the fourth floor, moderately isolated from others. We were able to play, eat and snuggle in another area of the huge old Victorian house. I appreciated that, rooming at the Ronald McDonald House, we were able to make good time in the morning to our early appointments at the CHP Pulmonology Clinic.

At home, there were numerous trips to the hospital for weekly lab tests while establishing Josh's normal levels. There were frequent chest x-rays to check the position of, and to clear the Broviac catheter of blood clots with Urokinase.[40] Our life became a whirlwind of CHP visits every month for clinic visits and lung biopsies, local lab draws, chest x-rays, local pediatrician appointments and frequent ER visits.

Months earlier, when I recognized that transplant was indeed becoming a reality for us, I began to do some research on lung transplantation. I located information which, alarmingly, describes a problem found in some lung transplant patients, Obliterative Bronchiolitis (OB).

I have often thought that my obsessive research may have been a mistake, but I've always been one who likes to be prepared and understand what to expect. Awareness of the OB issue made me only slightly familiar with it and only served to terrify me once we received that diagnosis following a lung biopsy just a few months post-transplant. Perhaps in some cases, ignorance *is* bliss?

---

[40] . An enzyme that is produced by the kidney and found in urine, that activates plasminogen, and that is used therapeutically to dissolve blood clots (as in the heart). – Merriam-Webster

CHAPTER 16

Long-Awaited Make-A-Wish

In October 1995, the Make-A-Wish NASCAR trip became a reality for Josh and his dad. On Friday, October 6th, they flew from Buffalo, New York to Charlotte, North Carolina where they rented a car and proceeded to their hotel. Josh's long-awaited dream was finally coming true!

At the track the next day, they met up with Cici, the Pittsburgh Make-A-Wish representative who had made this all happen. Josh was invited to the garage to meet his hero, Dale Earnhardt, Sr., to have pictures taken. There he was given a #3 hat autographed by his hero. The team owner Richard Childress and couple of crew members added their autographs to his cherished hat. Mr. Childress then took Josh to the driver's meeting to meet drivers and owners. This was a true honor for Josh as "outsiders" are not permitted into this meeting. Jan and Josh were invited into Jeff Bodine's hauler, talked with him, observing set-up of engines and parts and how that's all done. All exciting stuff for them!

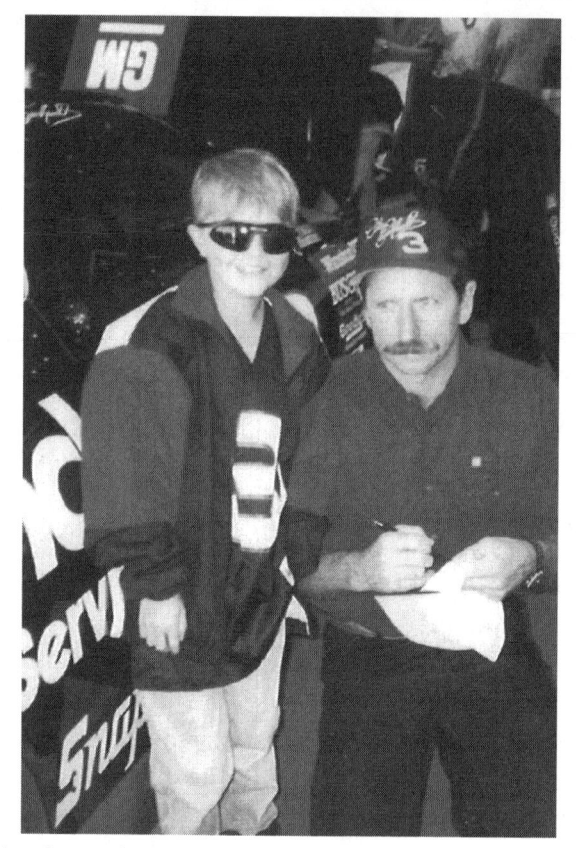

Josh and Dale Earnhardt, Sr. in the garage at Charlotte Motor Speedway on October 8, 1995. That smile says it all…Josh couldn't be happier!

Josh and his dad watched the Busch Race on Saturday, then on Sunday, Dale Earnhardt, Sr. raced in the Winston Cup. They had box seats and wore headsets so they were able to hear the commentators. That day, Earnhardt started the race last and finished second.

It warms my heart knowing that so many people did so much to ensure that Josh finally received his Make-A-Wish. A year or two following Josh's death I learned that at the Millcreek Mall in Erie, there would be a Make-A-Wish wind chime display. Every child who received a wish had their own chime. It took a while but I located Josh's chime. The chime only revealed his first name, his wish and the wish date. It was an enormously emotional trip, to say the least.

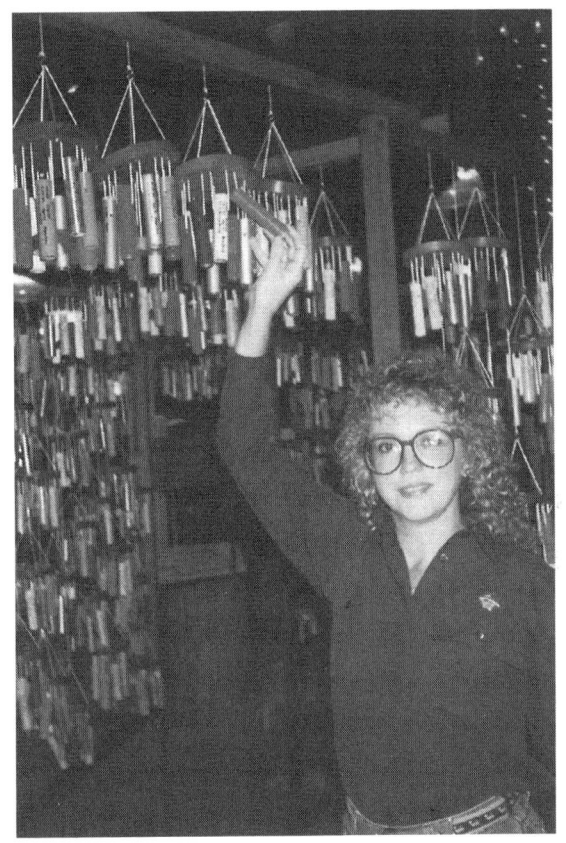

So many Make-A Wish Chimes!

    In the fall of 1996 when his dad let him drive his truck on a remote dirt road, all he could talk about was the used S-10 truck displayed prominently and for sale at a local Chevy dealership. He pointed the truck out to me every time we passed by on the way to Grammie's house. I was even excited for him, that he was nearly old enough to drive. He had something to look forward to and motivate him!

    The news of his favorite NASCAR driver, Dale Earnhardt's death on February 18, 2001 was distressing for me, knowing what an important person he had been in Josh's life. He had compassionately spent time with children whom he had never met before but had admired him from afar. My only consolation is that they are now 'up there' together as I envision Josh on his motorcycle and Dale in his #3 car.

CHAPTER 17

Chilling Experiences

The following data is gleaned from a letter to Dr. McConnell regarding our CHP appointments of December 28 and 29, 1995.

Josh showed a hard-earned weight gain (yippee!). No change was noted on his chest x-ray but crackles were heard in all the lung fields. Significant deterioration in his Pulmonary Function Tests were reported. A well-tolerated bronchoscopy and lung biopsy revealed inflammatory cells and lymphocytic bronchitis, considered to be a form of rejection. There was also pneumonitis consistent with a viral infection and CMV. The letter stated plans to discuss and revise Josh's treatment management.

Josh was subsequently admitted to CHP on January 11, 1996 for three days of high-dose IV Solu-Medrol (steroids) for treatment of rejection. That day's PFTs showed no improvement and there were even more crackles heard in both lung bases. He was also being treated with IV Ganciclovir, an antiviral medication. Not the first time, I thought, "How much can this little body take?"

As a fiercely vigilant advocate of my precious child, I was sleeping in Josh's room and doing my very best to fulfill my motherly obligation to drive a teenage boy crazy. I believe I was quite successful in my efforts. On the 13th we were allowed out on a pass, and it was a great relief for both of us to escape the confines of the hospital. We enjoyed local restaurants immensely, Josh ordering whatever he wanted. Pack those calories in!

God Bless Josh for being as patient as he was with this whole apparently unending process. I tried very hard, but generally unsuccessfully, not to stress over these mounting health issues, pushing negative thoughts to the back where I hoped they would not resurface. Fleetingly, thoughts would sometimes come forward about his growing number of school absences. I recognized that he was quickly falling behind others in his class. Yet, it was unexpected how rapidly school issues were dropping lower on the priority list. Let's just keep this child well.

Josh had tolerated his IV and other treatments very well. The frequent labs? Well, let's just say they were a continuous pain. Literally. Gratefully, Josh was discharged on the 14th with our instructions on tapering the steroid dose. Josh was cautioned to be alert for CMV esophagitis and we were to call immediately if there were any problems.

When you're struggling to find the energy just to walk around the house, what else can you be thinking about? Who wants to study when you can barely breathe? Lung associations all over the world agree, "When you can't breathe, nothing else matters". And in the end, that's really what it all comes down to.

January 25, 1996: back in Pittsburgh for repeat PFTs and a lung biopsy, review of Josh's chart reflects that after his last hospitalization he had been experiencing increasing anxiety, was depressed and had increased fears of dying. Even today, while reviewing his medical records, tears well up and I experience pain and anxiety reading about this. A child should not have to live with these fears.

We were informed that the lung biopsy would have to be repeated the next day, the 26th, in an attempt to determine the cause of the continued drop off in his Pulmonary Function Testing results. Oh, what pain in my heart for my precious baby. *Please, just let me trade places.*

Our next CHP visit was on February 14 and 15, 1996. Josh had a PFT and an exercise test. The exercise test entailed riding a bike and being hooked up with all kinds of wires and sensors to monitor his oxygen level, oxygen consumption, blood pressure, etc. Josh had poor exercise tolerance, as indicated by his "peak work rate" of 35% of predicted. His low exercise tolerance was thought to be attributed to ventilatory (lung) limitation, as well as peripheral limitations associated with severe physical deconditioning both prior to and following transplantation.

The PFT showed findings consistent with severe smaller airway obstruction with air trapping. In comparison with the exam on January 25, 1996, there was further deterioration in expiratory flow function and more air trapping. He was also showing abnormally low oxygen levels in room air. These were alarming findings to me, considering there was only a three-week interval between these PFTs. Is there no end to the worry? Just be careful what you wish for.

CHAPTER 18

Chicken Pox

On the evening of February, 16 1996, Josh began noticing one or two itchy spots on his scalp and by Saturday morning when he woke up, he had many more on his legs and body. We immediately went to a clinic at the hospital where his pediatrician was on duty; he sent him right to the ER. The doctors noted that he had rales, wheezing and a fever.[41][42] After a thorough examination, it was thought to be Varicella (Chicken Pox) causing the issues. After a telephone consult with one of the CHP pulmonologists, Josh was started on an IV antibiotic given over one hour, then we promptly proceeded to CHP.

Upon admission, he was put into a positive pressure isolation room.[43] This environment is used for patients with compromised immune systems, such as transplant recipients who are on immunosuppressant medications. Air will flow out of the room rather than in, so that any airborne bacteria that may infect the patient are kept outside the room. In order to maintain the positive pressure, the room is sealed utilizing a two-door airlock system.

---

[41] . Rales are abnormal lung sounds characterized by discontinuous clicking or rattling sounds. – easyauscultation.com

[42] . Wheezing is a high-pitched whistling sound made while breathing. It's often associated with difficulty breathing. Wheezing may occur during breathing out (expiration) or breathing in (inspiration). - Mayo Clinic

[43] . Hospitals may have positive pressure rooms for patients with compromised immune systems. Air will flow out of the room instead of in, so that any airborne microorganisms (e.g., bacteria) that may infect the patient are kept away. - Wikipedia

On the day of admission, Josh was tired and pale, had a 102° fever and was experiencing abdominal pain. Later that day he complained of two different occurrences of stabbing back pain on the right, along with a feeling of a "lump in his throat". It was found that he had Varicella lesions in his mouth and throat and due to this, he was less able to eat and drink due to the pain. A chest x-ray showed hyperinflation (over-inflation), of the lungs, increased interstitial markings, but thankfully, no pneumonia or atelectasis.[44]

On the 18th, after multiple painful attempts to obtain blood, Josh would not tolerate any more "sticks". The nurse noticed that he was becoming very anxious due to all the needle sticks and was beginning to hyperventilate. The lab tech said the bloodwork would be attempted again the next morning, that stick thankfully done successfully. There's always something you can find to be grateful for. Josh was given Cepacol™ lozenges for the sore throat, Aveeno™ baths and Calamine™ lotion for the itchy lesions. An Acyclovir (antiviral medication) IV was initiated to treat the Varicella virus.

February 19th charting reveals that Josh was not in good spirits. His temperature was over 102°, and he had been having occasional vomiting. Oddly, the vomiting did seem to ease the abdominal pain for a time. It seems to me fairly reasonable that anyone feeling this way would be justified in failing to be sweet and sociable. The abdominal pain was felt to be mild hepatitis secondary to the varicella infection.

The morning of February 20th, Josh stated that he was, as he said, "feeling lousy", was even more tender in the right upper abdomen when examined by the consulting Infectious Disease MD, presumably due to the mild hepatitis. After following up on the Liver Function Test, the Infectious Disease physician agreed with the pulmonologist that an ultrasound of the right upper quadrant, specifically the liver, should be done. In addition, new lesions had appeared on his back. Increased wheezes and crackles were noted in both lungs. During these difficult days, the only entertainment Josh could tolerate was watching some TV in between restless naps.

The Acyclovir IV was to continue as long as there were new Varicella lesions appearing. A nurse's note on the chart on the 20th states that "still new lesions despite Acyclovir", raises the question in my mind that normally with use of this treatment, the lesions should have been diminishing by

---

[44] . A complete or partial collapse of the entire lung or area (lobe) of the lung. – Mayo Clinic

then. Due to this lack of response to treatment, the physicians opted to initiate a temporary reduction of Josh's immunosuppression drugs that would promote a more normal immune response to the virus while treatment of the active varicella was taking place.

Josh had also been placed on Bactrim and Augmentin for a probable sinus infection and was given Benadryl in combination with Maalox for the throat pain. The pulmonologist's chart notes from the morning of the 21st state that Josh was feeling much better, was smiling and was in general good spirits. He was experiencing decreased abdominal pain. There were no new lesions and no fever. His chest exam sounded better with no wheezes. Seen simultaneously by the Infectious Disease (ID) physician, he suggested that the Acyclovir be continued for the rest of the day and also recommended following the lesions to assure there were no new ones.

Per the Infectious Disease physician, the isolation as well as the Acyclovir might be discontinued the next day, the 22nd; he would see Josh the next morning and make that determination at that time. The next day there were still two lesions that were not yet scabbed, so the decision was made to keep him in isolation and remain on Acyclovir. Other children in the hospital could not be exposed to Varicella if he was transported throughout the hospital still presenting with active lesions. Considering continued crackles and wheezes heard in the lungs, the pulmonologist also suggested a CT of the chest be done at the same time as the head and neck scans which had already been ordered.

It seemed we had finally turned a corner. What a balancing act this whole admission had been. Unfortunately, lab draws were frequent but necessary. They were done to closely monitor Josh's FK—immunosuppressant—and creatinine levels.[45]

On the 22nd, the Pulmonary/Nutrition Dietician followed up on her initial evaluation that was done on February 19, 1996. She noted that he was in good spirits, his appetite was improving, he was having no pain swallowing and no stomach pain. She also wrote on the chart that Josh was reluctant to take the supplements. She gave him an alternative menu selection list and encouraged him to increase his intake, an admittedly

---

[45] . Creatinine is a chemical waste product that's produced by your muscle metabolism and to a smaller extent by eating meat. Healthy kidneys filter creatinine and other waste products from your blood. The filtered waste products leave your body in your urine. – Mayo Clinic

difficult task when your stomach is compressed by hyperinflated lungs. To better track weight gain/loss from this point on, she asked that Josh be weighed before discharge and asked the physicians to consider ordering labs for PT time (Prothrombin, or clotting time). The ID doctor noted that the Varicella lesions were finally resolving and that all were scabbed. It was finally OK to discontinue isolation as well as the Acyclovir therapy.

On the morning of the 23rd, Josh was feeling markedly better. He was released from isolation to a regular room on the floor, a delightful development. Fortunately, his albumin findings were improved.[46] An Ear, Nose and Throat (ENT) consult had been suggested.

After active infection, when all lesions were crusted over, a chest x-ray was recommended to check for bronchiectasis.[47] As there continued to be crackles in his lungs, all three CT Scans were performed on the 23rd. These exams were ordered because some of the lab test results were consistent with an active infection. There also was interest in ruling out sinus polyps due to a runny nose and chronic nasal congestion lasting for several years.

February 24th: Josh had no complaints; the Varicella rash was still improving and his Albumin level continued to improve. The normal FK dose was resumed, and levels were to be watched closely via the labs which would be drawn the next morning. Josh was feeling better; in order to pass the time, we played cards and other games, watched TV, made phone calls and otherwise entertained ourselves, feeling optimistic with the recent positive turn of events.

February 25th: Josh did well overnight; his blood pressure and respirations were good. Labs to recheck current medication levels were drawn. However, it was noted that there were persistently abnormal chest x-rays, and his symptoms of clear watery nasal discharge were continuous. The Infectious Disease doctor had noted in the chart, referring to the initial Sinus CT report, that there were dramatic findings for pansinusitis, worse

---

[46] . An albumin blood test measures the amount of albumin in your blood. Albumin is a protein made by your liver. Albumin helps keep fluid in your bloodstream so it doesn't leak into other tissues. It is also carries various substances throughout your body, including hormones, vitamins, and enzymes. Low albumin levels can indicate a problem with your liver or kidneys. – MedlinePlus

[47] . Bronchiectasis: Permanent abnormal widening of the bronchi (air tubes that branch deep into the lungs). Bronchiectasis can cause recurrent lung infections, a disabling cough, shortness of breath, and coughing up blood. - MedicineNet

on the left than the right.[48] She suspected non-allergic rhinitis (a set of symptoms that resemble an allergy but that occur without a known cause producing symptoms such as postnasal drip, runny nose, sneezing).[49] There was also blurring of some of the bones surrounding the ethmoid sinuses, likely related to mucosal turbinate hypertrophy (increase in the volume of an organ or tissue due to the enlargement of its component cells).[50]

Finally discharged on the 25th of February with adjusted meds, we had been in CHP for an arduous and, for the most part, quite unpleasant nine-day admission. It had certainly felt so much longer than that, being sequestered for the majority of the time in one room that seemed to become smaller every day.

---

[48] . Inflammation of all the accessory sinuses of the nose on one or both sides. - MediLexicon

[49] . Inflammation of the nasal mucous membrane. - MediLexicon

[50] . The nasal turbinates are long, narrow passageways that help to warm and moisten the air that flows in through the nose. The turbinates are also called the nasal conchae. If the turbinates are too large, they can actually block airflow. Doctors call this condition turbinate hypertrophy. - Healthline

CHAPTER 19

Additional Health Issues

On February 29, 1996, just days after discharge, Josh had yet another a lung biopsy with a CHP hospital admission for observation. A set of PFTs showed decreased function.

Since his February 25th discharge, Josh hadn't felt well, noticed decreased energy and was experiencing a decrease in his spirometry numbers. He had been using his Proventil inhaler every 45 minutes to get relief. Spirometry is an easy test we had started doing and documenting at home, using a small easily utilized device.[51]

On 1 liter of oxygen, the pulse oximetry numbers for the first five days of admission remained in the high 80s to the low 90s. By the 4th of March, it had improved, varying anywhere from 96-100%.

The chart notes that there were multiple healing Chicken Pox lesions and healed scars. There was a significant change in the chest x-ray and lung exam since the last visit, and Josh appeared ill. It showed opacities that had increased since the previous films of February 29, 1996. Findings were suggestive of pneumonia and multiple cystic changes throughout the lungs.

---

[51] . Spirometry (spy-ROM-uh-tree) is a common office test used to assess how well your lungs work by measuring how much air you inhale, how much you exhale and how quickly you exhale. Spirometry is used to diagnose asthma, chronic obstructive pulmonary disease (COPD) and other conditions that affect breathing. – Mayo Clinic

There were multiple suppositions as to why there would be this extreme change in only a few days, and the BAL should provide some clues as to the diagnosis.[52] Labwork following the biopsy revealed that CMV was present.

The Pulmonary Nutritionist noted that Josh's appetite and intake remained poor. Josh had lost about four and a half pounds in the past two weeks resulting in nutritional risk. She encouraged fluids and oral intake and that weight be checked twice a week. A very gradual improvement was noted over the next few days.

A chest x-ray done on March 5th showed that there was a decrease in the degree of interstitial lung markings since the prior study, showing resolving edema (swelling from fluid) and/or rejection.[53] The attending physician noted that Josh continued to show improvement, and steroid doses he was receiving were only "asthma" doses. Josh was finally discharged on March 8th with plans to return on the 13th for a follow-up Pulmonary appointment.

My review of Josh's medical records for the purpose of writing this book brought back long-forgotten pain, heartache and distress reading about all of the abnormalities and complications found on the biopsy as well as the physicians' examinations. Test results and physician observations reflected persistent decrease in lung function, weight and general health.

---

[52] . Bronchoalveolar lavage; BAL; informally, "bronchoalveolar washing", is a medical procedure in which a bronchoscope is passed through the mouth or nose into the lungs and fluid is squirted into a small part of the lung and then collected for examination. - Wikipedia

[53] . Relating to or situated in the small, narrow spaces between tissues or parts of an organ: interstitial cells; interstitial fluid. – Your Dictionary

CHAPTER 20

A Year Following Transplant

In mid-August, 1996, we again ended up in the ER, this time Josh's mediport in his left thigh was blocked and needed a saline and heparin flush followed by labwork. We repeated this procedure in the ER in early October and again in early November.

As a Junior Volunteer at Warren General Hospital, Josh, though working in the Snack Bar, had initially wanted to work during the summer months transporting patients to and from Imaging Services where I worked. Ultimately, he recognized that he was currently physically unable to handle the challenges of the task. I later received numerous comments from various hospital employees about his positive attitude, good manners and courtesy toward customers and fellow volunteers. I recognize that I must have done something right!

In July of 1996, I hosted a picnic for family and friends and ordered a cake to celebrate the first anniversary of Josh's "second chance" at life and double-lung transplant. I laughed when I saw the lungs on the cake were positioned upside-down, but this did not at all dampen the festivities. It was undoubtedly a milestone to remember, an additional year of fully enjoying life.

A year after transplant, Josh was able to join a baseball team. His small stature at fourteen years in comparison to his peers was the result of his chronic lung disease. I recall him being advised to crouch a little, making his strike zone even smaller. It was difficult for him to run fast enough to make it to first base but walking him helped to keep him in the game. Caring, kind and compassionate coach and team members made for great memories!

Having a small mouth, Josh's teeth were crowded and in serious need of straightening. He had braces applied and each month chose varied colors that were important to him: Earnhardt, Pirates, Buffalo Bills, revealing his diverse allegiances. He made each experience as creative and interesting as possible. He was also pleased to be able to play touch football with friends in one of the city parks, something that helped him further feel part of a group and "one of the guys".

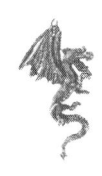

CHAPTER 21

Many Additional Medical Problems Cropping Up

On November 28, 1996, we were on our way home from a clinic visit and we stopped at his favorite restaurant, Chi Chi's. It was Josh's 15th birthday and I had arranged for a birthday cake and the wait staff to sing to him.

There were increasingly frequent CHP Pulmonary Clinic appointments as time went on. We accumulated many waiting room hours, talking, laughing and figuring out how to pleasantly pass the time.

The CHP Endocrinology Department was following him as his growth had always been slow, in part, secondary to chronic steroid use, as well as from burning so many calories merely through the struggle of breathing. Supplemental nutrition was recommended by the Nutrition Department in order to maintain an acceptable weight, a tall order for Josh. He was being bombarded from all sides. A Pulmonology Nutritionist was also following Josh, as he was having difficulty maintaining weight, let alone gaining.

On January 23, 1997, a CHP transbronchial biopsy revealed acute cellular rejection in addition to acute and chronic bronchitis.[54] A week later Josh was admitted to Warren General Hospital for three days to receive three IV doses of steroids delivered through his mediport. Due to this treatment, his heart rate increased and blood pressure was very low. There would be continual monitoring of his vitals and labwork to watch for low levels of potassium. Pre-treatment labs were drawn to

---

[54] . Bronchoscopy with transbronchial biopsy is a procedure in which a bronchoscope is inserted through the nose or mouth to collect several pieces of lung tissue. – UCLA Health

establish his baseline electrolytes and liver functions; post-treatment (he was experiencing steroid-induced diabetes), there would be follow-ups to assure all was returning to normal.

I often prayed that it could be me. A child should not have to live with this experience. I sometimes wonder what he thought of his life, his chronic health issues, if he wished he could be like other kids, to be normal and healthy. Did his heart ache for that, as mine did?

We were back in our ER bright and early on February 4, 1997, Josh with a fever of 101°. After an exam and results of Josh's labwork were returned (all were found to be elevated), a CHP pulmonologist was consulted and he requested that we proceed to CHP immediately. By the time we arrived, the fever had increased to 103° and his heart rate was 132 and blood pressure elevated. He was experiencing possible sepsis and rejection of his double-lung transplant, complicated by Bronchiolitis Obliterans.

The next day it was determined that Josh's immunosuppression with Imuran would be continued, but he was also started on what was then known as FK506[55], along with a bolus of IV fluids to stabilize his blood pressure. [56]) High doses of IV steroids were begun to treat the acute rejection[57]. IV fluids were maintained after the bolus was completed.

Epstein-Barr Virus (EBV), identified on Josh's lab tests, is of great significance in transplant recipients. Most likely contracted from his donor, EBV is a major complication of transplant recipients. This virus raised its ugly head again during this admission. It was learned that the WGH blood cultures done in the ER on the 4th were positive for Staph. Josh was immediately put on a 10-day course of antibiotics.

By the next morning, Josh's fever was lower, he reported no chills and stated that he felt better than yesterday. His heart rate and blood pressure were somewhat improved, and he was breathing with less difficulty.

---

[55] . Tacrolimus, also known as fujimycin or FK506, is an immunosuppressive drug used mainly after allogeneic organ transplant to lower the risk of organ rejection.
[56] . Bolus: a: a dose of a substance (such as a drug) given intravenously, b: a large dose of a substance given by injection for the purpose of rapidly achieving the needed therapeutic concentration in the bloodstream dose of a substance (such as a drug) given intravenously. – Merriam-Webster
[57] . Transplant rejection occurs when transplanted tissue is rejected by the recipient's immune system, which destroys the transplanted tissue. Transplant rejection can be lessened by determining the molecular similitude between donor and recipient and by use of immunosuppressant drugs after transplant. - Wikipedia

Although his oxygen requirement was lower, his vital signs continued to be closely monitored and aerosol treatments continued. Although his chest x-rays continued to show improvement, decreasing crackles and wheezes were noted. The attending physician had stated that Josh was only receiving "asthma therapy" doses of steroids.

However, the Pulmonary Nutritionist noted on the chart that Josh's appetite and intake were poor and his weight was down by almost four and a half pounds since the 17th of February and was currently at nutritional risk. She again recommended his weight be checked twice a week.

Nurses chart notes showed that on the 6th, although he still had a low fever, Josh felt better, but was upset that he had to be in Pittsburgh. He stated that when possible, he preferred to be at Warren General Hospital, closer to home, friends and family. On this day, it was found via an Ultrasound exam that there was a clot in his mediport causing swelling in his leg. Repeated Urokinase infusions into the Mediport failed to dissolve the clot. When are we going to get a break?

February 8th found us out of the hospital on a pass, a much-needed respite from hospital life. We always enjoyed these passes, a break from hospital life which was becoming depressing.

On the 10th repeat PFTs were performed, showing improvement of the values found back on January 27. An ultrasound of the mediport in his pelvis, obtained on the same day, confirmed a thrombus (blood clot), and blood flow into his leg was found to be solely through collateral veins. The mediport was removed in Surgery the next day without complication, and he continued on antibiotics.

Thankfully, Josh was feeling great on Thursday, February 13th, and he pressured his docs to let him go home; I guess he figured he'd been patient enough (no pun intended). Sensing there was something more to the story than he was saying, they asked why he was so anxious to get out of the hospital. With a somewhat self-conscious grin, he confessed that he had planned to go to a Valentine's Day dance (with a girl!) on Friday night. Of course, they felt obligated to tease him about it, but delightedly got on board with his plan since he was improved, and discharged him the next morning, as his treatment was complete by that time.

In the afternoon, we made a trip to the florist to buy a big bunch of carnations for Josh's special first—and only—date. It was exciting to watch him in the floral shop contemplating the numerous varieties and colors of flowers, trying to make a decision. This event was almost as thrilling for me as it was for him.

On March 7, 1997, there was another three-day CHP admission for an additional round of high-dose IV immunosuppression therapy along with IV Ganciclovir, intended to slow the growth and spread of Josh's CMV. Again, his blood pressure, electrolytes and blood sugar were closely monitored. He had a Modified Barium Swallow to rule out aspiration as the cause of his current problems.

On the morning of March 24th, Josh wasn't feeling well and was unable to attend school. I called him throughout the day to check on him, and he'd say he just wasn't feeling well. Arriving home at the end of the workday, I learned that he was being alarmingly stoic; I could see that his situation had become very worrisome. I had to practically carry him to the car and zoomed off to the pediatrician's office. From there, after checking blood pressure, oxygen Sats and other vital signs, they conferred with Pittsburgh pulmonologists, and an ambulance took him to WGH. The pulmonologists had immediately arranged for a helicopter to pick Josh up at the hospital.

Josh was septic, a life-threatening situation. My thoughts immediately were guilty, "Oh, why didn't I go home at lunch to check on him?" In the ER, after what seemed an eternity, the Pittsburgh helicopter crew arrived. They wrapped him in a foil blanket and tucked him in on the stretcher. They distracted him by talking about the Hale-Bopp comet being visible and told him he'd be able to watch it from the chopper on the way to Pittsburgh.

Watching that helicopter take off, my heart sunk to an all-time low while my anxiety flew in the opposite direction. I was looking at a lonely, seemingly interminable three-hour trip before I learned if my son had survived. I had called Jan and we both found our way to CHP. This was an enormously difficult and emotional trip, worse than any other; the drive to Pittsburgh for transplant not even a close second.

I remember with chilling clarity the ICU physician telling Jan and me when we finally arrived, that Josh was on a ventilator and the situation was "touch and go"; there were no guarantees as to the outcome. An appropriately vague statement, I suppose, for parents facing the imminent death of their only child. Prayer was our only option at this point. We were both terrified to the very core; I couldn't eat or sleep, my mind scattered, going in a million different directions. How did I even find my way down here?

We shared a tiny parent's room with two cots, unable to sleep, we just rested as much as possible. Two days into this hospital admission, as he was still on a ventilator in ICU, I sat by Josh's bed holding his hand, brushing his hair (which he had always loved because it was so relaxing to him), talking to him and playing his favorite country music tapes. Glancing at the tubing between his catheter and urine bag, I was shocked to see a quantity of white material in his urine. I asked the nurse if this indicated a bladder or kidney infection.

This is merely confirmation to parents out there that you must keep your eyes and ears open, be observant and be your loved one's advocate. Ask the questions and point out any difficulties you feel your loved one may be having. Be alert to the progression of his or her illness and their care. If you have that nagging little voice in the back of your head, there is a reason--ask the questions, as inconsequential as they may seem.

The nurse got to work right away, sending a urine sample to the Lab for analysis. Of course, it was an eternity in my mind before testing was completed and the results were available. I was right, there was a big-time infection in progress and treatment began immediately. It was pure torture to watch the nurse introduce an antibiotic solution directly into Josh's bladder through the catheter to treat the infection. Even on the ventilator and heavily medicated, he fought and squirmed in his bed, visibly in a great deal of discomfort. This was just painful to witness.

The next day while being weaned from the ventilator, and on a lower dose of meds, Josh was starting to tug at his endotracheal tube. I thought that because his meds were lighter he was fighting the tube, but through nearly indecipherable notes, at last I learned that the tube was causing his braces to embed in his cheek, causing him a great deal of discomfort. He had been merely trying to move the tubing to decrease the pressure on his mouth. I remember his frustration trying to communicate this to me, as well as his confusion and difficulty trying to write a note about it while still on heavy meds. My heart just aches for him as these memories come painfully flooding back in waves.

A couple attempts were required to get him weaned from the ventilator, as his oxygen Sats were not improving as we had hoped. This was very frightening to observe, wondering whether he would eventually be able to breathe on his own. It was such a difficult admission for him and enormously stressful for us. The ventilator had been breathing for him for three days; now he would have to remember how to breathe on his own.

Later when Josh was weaned from the ventilator, he described specific things that had happened and what he had heard while he was on the ventilator. During the time a patient is on a ventilator, they are given medications so that they are unaware or experience amnesic effects. Josh's recollections during this time period, however, were confirmed by an RN.

I found that I had an irritation of one of my eyes the whole time we were in Pittsburgh, apparently blown in when I was watching the helicopter depart. While still at CHP, I called home to make an appointment for an eye examination when I got home. It was definitely low on my priority list, but during the whole time there, that little something would annoy me, a very trivial thing considering recent events, but was something that would eventually need to be addressed.

So, when we finally—and joyfully—returned home, I kept my eye appointment and gratefully had a foreign body removed. As I returned home wearing an eye patch, Josh saw me, chuckled, and disappeared into his room for a moment and emerged with Paul Parrot. He plopped Paul onto my shoulder and said in his best pirate inflection, "Aargh! Here's your parrot, Long John Silver."

I've come to realize how appropriate Josh's name is. According to the dictionary, to "josh" means to tease [someone] in a playful way; it can also suggest good-natured banter. His personality certainly fostered his name. I have learned to savor every delicious moment of his life with love and respect.

As I sit here today at the keyboard, I look wistfully at Paul, watching me from his perch on my desk beside drowsy Omar II and reflect on how amazingly young-looking Paul is at 38 years old. I smile lovingly at the heart-warming memory of Josh's characteristic chuckle and humor.

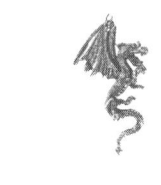

CHAPTER 22

Struggling to Start Life Over

My good friend Stacy had mentioned at lunch on a Thursday in late April of 1997 that she had seen a personal ad in the newspaper. A man named Ken was looking for someone to golf with. I asked her if she was crazy! Didn't she know what lunatics there were out there? After thinking about this conversation for a day, on Friday night after work, Josh at his dad's, I called just to listen to this guy's recorded message. Holy cow, what a deep, sexy voice!

I thought about this overnight then left Ken a message on Saturday morning. Later that day he returned my call, we talked for a while and arranged to meet at a local golf course where we agreed to play a round. What a light in my life he proved to be, especially at this dreadful phase of my life. This was the man who would eventually become my husband.

Ken met Josh a few days later and commented on his initiative for hosing the dirt out of the garage. I was so proud that Josh was recognized for his motivation, enthusiasm and incentive. How lucky I was to have this wonderful son! We all went inside and watched and discussed NASCAR; Josh liked Ken immediately. I was not prepared for what just two weeks in the future held in store.

Jan had taken Josh to his May CHP Pulmonology Clinic appointment, as I had burned through the remainder of my vacation with the lengthy February CHP stay. But before they even returned home, both his Transplant Coordinator and Dr. Kurland called me to give me a heads-up. In essence, they said that Josh was yet again at *end-stage disease* (words that send a chill down my spine even now) and was immediately placed back on the transplant list.

Dr. Kurland had asked Josh, "Are you mad at me?" because he was very quiet after this was announced. Josh's subdued response was, "No, I'm just disappointed." We cried together when he got home and I suggested we take the Blazer and go drive off Niagara Falls together. After sharing a brief laugh at this outrageous statement, we sat and rocked and held each other. I couldn't imagine how I could possibly watch this precious child endure another transplant. Surely, he was secretly pondering the same thing.

Josh was experiencing extreme shortness of breath in the morning of May 13th and our breathing treatments at home didn't seem to help. We went to the WGH ER early that morning; I called Jan, and he came to be with us during this worrisome time. Following review of the results of a portable chest x-ray and various lab tests, the WGH physicians were in contact with a CHP pulmonologist for guidance. The breathing treatments and other meds finally brought Josh into his comfort zone, so we went back home, very relieved that we'd once again dodged the bullet.

Wednesday, May 14, 1997: the following sequence of events is forever imprinted in my memory. Here is where many times I have had to click "Save", closed the manuscript document and not return for months at a time. The time surrounding the emotional transplant experience was extremely difficult for me to write about, but I found that it was infinitely more challenging to relate this horrendous part of our story.

This morning brought the same circumstances as the day before. The breathing treatments at home again were not helping. Again, I called his dad to the ER. There were more labs, another portable chest x-ray and significantly more apprehension and anxiety on my part. My strength and courage were rapidly eroding with each passing minute. Josh was leaning on a bedside table in an ER exam room, his shoulders elevated, struggling to draw each breath. Terrified, my heart practically pounded out of my chest. Again, I was seeing that look that I'd glimpsed once before, nearly two years prior in the CHP ICU a couple days following transplant. Josh had been in extreme pain and asked me with a terrified look on his face if he was going to die. Now at fifteen and a half years old, the question remained unspoken, but I read it in his eyes. On this morning, I could see that he already knew the answer. When I saw this, I was terrified as never before. Painfully, I relived it all as I wrote these lines.

Cindy, his old friend, a Respiratory Therapist, stayed in the exam room with him as I left. Through endless PFTs and breathing treatments, for several years they had been teasing each other back and forth good-naturedly about their respective favorite NASCAR drivers. It would be many months later that she would tell me that when I left the room that day, he pleaded with her, "Please don't tell my mom. I don't want her to cry." Yes, *he knew*. I can't fully describe the horror, the pain and the disbelief I still feel to this day, aware that my child knew these were the last minutes of his life here on this Earth.

He was exhausted – physically, mentally, emotionally. He could take no more. It was obvious when I looked in his eyes. His look of acceptance and resignation before I left the room instantly sent terror, never before known, down into the depths of my soul. It was the look of a final "goodbye". This image is forever seared in my brain. A blackness pushed forward by the dread sat heavily on my heart. With high anxiety, I went to the ER nurse's desk and called Dr. Kurland in Pittsburgh to beg that a helicopter be sent STAT. God bless him, he was going to make it happen. I felt confident that again, as yesterday, he would be feeling better, breathing easier, as relief immediately washed over me, confident that we would pull Josh back from the brink of death once more.

Meanwhile, seeing his severe distress, the staff had already moved Josh from the exam room into a regular ER room by the time I had completed the call. I barged right in and saw a nurse, respiratory technician and anesthesiologist working on him. There was something wrong on the heart monitor. Josh was looking at me while I was told he was going to be sedated, intubated and placed on a ventilator. He was OK with this; it was now a familiar experience, and it would be a welcome relief from this struggle. I was asked to step out of the room, so I gave him a quick kiss and a weak smile, telling him I loved him and it was going to be OK. By now I had totally panicked, standing outside the door, listening as my knees shook, becoming increasingly alarmed and unsteady on my feet.

The nursing supervisor, knowing Stacy and I were close, had tried to call her so she could be with me. I recall Stacy telling me later that because her phone line was busy the operator had to break in to reach her. In her panic, she couldn't find her car keys; when she finally located them, she sped to the hospital, ignoring speed limits.

I was guided away from the door in a daze, terrified, looking for someone, anyone to hold onto. Someone led me out of the ER into the waiting room. I was crying; friends from my department, Imaging, and other departments had come to check on us both and attempted to comfort me. I couldn't think straight; all I could do was sit, not knowing where to go, what to do, what to say, how to help, what exactly to pray.

I was then led to the Family Room where Jan had finally arrived. I have no sense of time during this dream-like morning, but the nursing supervisor returned a few minutes later and said to us, "It doesn't look good." Those words went straight to my heart like an arrow. They haunted me for a long time. I don't blame her for saying them, it's just that it is devastating statement for a parent to hear. There are no words that can cushion this event. I have a memory of saying, "No! I can't do this!" She left Jan and me alone. ALONE.

In that moment, that single suspended-in-time, slow-motion, horrific moment, my whole life changed forever. I lost my only child, my reason for being, my purpose, the meaning of my life. It simply couldn't be possible to survive this loss. God hadn't seen us through all these trials and tribulations just to end up here like this, had He? No! No, no, no!

Minutes later, it seemed we were in a time warp experiencing the worst pain a parent can imagine. I heard the nurse talking to Stacy outside the Family Room. They were speaking in muted tones, as if in a far-away dream, her words punctuated by Stacy's screaming when presented with the news.

The continual betrayal of an unhealthy body had brought us to this very day, this very moment. Josh had beaten back the dragon of this disease year after year until ultimately, no longer was his exhausted little body able to draw another agonized breath. His heart finally gave up the ultimate battle. He was gone. It was a parent's worst nightmare, like trying to run away from the monster (dragon) through deep, thick mud in a very, *very* bad dream. I prayed that I would wake up now, because I knew this could not be true.

Well, apparently it was, for we were led back into the ER room to be with Josh; I held his hand, rearranged his hair and noticed that his skin was becoming cool and mottled. "Dear God, let me die right here and now!" The words were screaming only in my head, but I wanted so badly to shout it to the world. I couldn't imagine leaving our child alone, unprotected. After all, this was my purpose in life. How could I ever turn my back and walk out? Can I be strong enough to survive this? So many questions, so few answers.

It is the worst feeling on earth for a parent to stand helpless beside a chronically ill child at the beginning of his life as well as at the end. We feel guilty because we are unable to change the circumstances, to help him, to save him because, well, that *is* a parent's job, right?

A nurse softly spoke to us, asking if we wanted an autopsy. Not even thinking of the procedure to soon take place in the funeral home, I was adamant that this not be done as Josh had endured enough "procedures" in his short life. In retrospect, I feel this was a mistake, a decision based solely on emotion. What could have been gleaned regarding Josh's disease might have helped future lung disease patients and transplant recipients. There is no turning back on the decision. I will always regret that.

We were asked whether we wanted to donate his corneas. Since he had suffered heart death, these were the only tissues that were now viable. That absolutely was a no-brainer. I knew for sure that Josh, more than being an organ recipient, would have also wanted to give the Gift of Life in the same spirit of generosity that had been shown him. He could now at least give the gift of sight. Jan and I agreed to it immediately. I have a wonderful letter from Upstate New York Transplant Services (UNYTS) which says, in part, "Though your concern for others during a time of personal grief, a three-month-old baby boy who was born blind was given the precious gift of sight." How incredibly rewarding it is to know that a part of Josh lives on enhancing another child's life!

Sensei Rick came into the room to console us. Chaplain Marcus Briggs kept us company and offered comfort as best he could; time passed in a flash. A nurse finally came to remind us that we were running out of time if we still wanted to donate his corneas. This final parting from Josh was so incredibly difficult.

In a daze and on a surreal mission, Jan and I left the hospital and drove together to the florist and then to the funeral home, both visits unbelievably excruciating. There were horribly difficult decisions that had to be made quickly about flowers, funeral home, obituary, casket, vault and headstone. It was all but impossible to focus on these pressing issues, but no procrastinating was permitted now. My heart hurt, my chest ached; how could I go on without this precious joking, smiling, chuckling, beautiful person?

On the unbearable drive back to an abruptly empty home, I was absolutely astounded how everyone was going on with their care-free lives. Really, hadn't the world just fallen off its axis? I couldn't get past the fact that Josh had been sitting next to me just three hours before, talking to me about how he was feeling, taking his breathing treatment, and asking to go to the hospital.

At that time, a beeper was the only means of contacting the transplant candidate if they weren't at home waiting by their phone. That day, upon arriving home, I found a package on the doorstep delivered by FedEx, a beeper to call Josh for his next transplant. There were so many things ripping my heart out! Was this a sign of the times to come?

At home, everywhere I looked there were fresh memories and relentless pain. My heart cried out in disbelief that he could have been in this room this morning and gone before 10 a.m.

When it was announced at school that morning that Josh had died, his friend Shawn later related to me that his entire class was dismissed; some of Josh's close friends needed even more time off. It is a tribute to Josh's memory that so many people thought so much of him. I am so very grateful that several have shared their thoughts and memories of him with me. I sense that many others saw inside the pure soul with which he walked, head held high, through his abbreviated, tormented life.

Regardless of age, the loss of a child is a violation of the normal order of life from which some never recover. The experience severely insults the sensibilities of loved ones, whether friends or family.

CHAPTER 23

A Thick Black Veil Falls

I was holding my son this morning and in one short hour was suddenly and unwillingly thrust into the unfamiliar, agonizing world of making funeral arrangements, choosing flowers, deciding which casket was the right one, discussing the obituary, picking out clothes to dress Josh in. What? He doesn't need shoes? This was strangeness over the top of the very uppermost top. I'd never imagined being in this position, having to make these decisions, to talk about my son in the past tense. What *is* this place? I was stuck in a spot in between life and this other "darkness" where I was lost and didn't know how to find the way out.

This was so surreal and certainly couldn't be true. I was sure I would wake up in the morning and our normal would have returned. But I could not sleep a wink that night, could not eat, though I tried to drink water. I was hearing the echoes of our laughter, seeing him in my mind; I was desperately lonely, disbelieving and in total, unrelenting agony. This was not real! Denial became my survival mode for a time. "Wait, *wait*…what just happened?" The unthinkable had become a cruel reality, my life, agonizing and unlivable. All I needed, all I wanted, was to see Josh's smiling face, to hear his voice (What? I can't remember his voice?), his chuckle, to trade places; please dear God, let it be me instead! Surely this is any parents' plea to God.

The fact of the matter is that men and women deal with the death of a child very differently. Dads many times feel they have to appear courageous for the family. They return to work and bury the grief deep inside so no one can see and feel that they have to be the strong one. Their grief eats them up from the inside. Moms do the "should have, could have, would have". Some leave the child's bedroom untouched, allowing no one to disturb personal items, while others get rid of anything that would serve as a painful reminder. I guess I fell somewhere in between. I gripped his things, clothing, toys, get well cards, just trying to catch his scent from everything in his room.

A great deal of misdirected guilt seems to accompany the helplessness. I have since learned that guilt is a universal reaction for grieving parents and that a very high percentage of marriages end in divorce following the loss of a child. Well, it had to be someone's fault, right? Although it is so easy to blame the other parent, that did not happen to us.

It was an eternity between May 14th and 17th, and an additional eternity before his headstone was put into place. Feeling lost with nothing to hold onto, I lived in an alternate reality where one minute I was in unbelievable pain and the next in a total fog, not knowing what to do or say next.

Jan and I stood together in Josh's room on the afternoon of Saturday May 17, 1997, following his funeral and after all the kind guests had departed, simply *looking*. The quiet in the house was absolutely deafening. We were so desolate, yet his spirit was there; I could feel him with me, trying to console us. In his closet were clothes I had just purchased for him the weekend before, tags still attached.

Josh's letter jacket was hanging there, huge on his little body, yet a great source of pride, as he was on the school's bowling team. His eight-pound fluorescent orange bowling ball inscribed with his name and a dragon was here. Hundreds of get-well and welcome home greeting cards were stacked neatly in a basket, keepsakes treasured and saved from the transplant nearly two years before; his dragon ring, dragon pendant, letters from and a picture of his amazing second cousin, Craig, whom he had respected and loved.

There were his most coveted belongings: cowboy boots with silver tips on the toes and spurs, a black duster, all cowboy gear acquired while in Albuquerque a few years before. His multiple karate gis, black belt, hakama and a variety of practice weapons used in his Shotokan Karate class were there, waiting to be taken up again. What was I to do? I prayed, "Dear God, please take me up into heaven also!" The pain was completely unbearable.

Walking into the kitchen, I saw the potted miniature pink rose Josh had given me for Mother's Day just last Sunday. Suddenly I recalled, "He has no school picture from this year! What will they put in the yearbook?" We had been on one of our emergency CHP trips when school pictures had been taken that year. It seemed strange that this peculiar thought would come into my head at that time, but apparently, this is typical of the scattered thoughts abounding while suffering recent grief. OK, already I could see that this was going to be infinitely miserable for a long, long time.

Though I was not the type who closed and locked up his room never to change a thing, it did take me a few years to finally let go of the loving cards and letters that Josh had received from friends and family in the hospital after his transplant. The sympathy cards that had poured in after his death, even from people we didn't know, were kept even longer. I almost felt as if I would be disposing of his memory if I got rid of these precious and heartfelt mementos.

It was difficult to give his things away; I likened it to giving a precious piece of him away. In the beginning, I clung to what was his, but eventually realized that others might appreciate and value some of his belongings. Many were given to my dear cousin's grandson, Joe, who was younger and adored and looked up to Josh.

Make-A-Wish called the week following Josh's death, with another offer for a NASCAR event, due to his re-listing for transplant. They were shocked to hear the news of his death. I was placed back into that dark whirlpool of repeated reminders.

Pittsburgh Children's Hospital routinely hosts a memorial service for their patients who have passed, and we attended one about a month after Josh's death. Before the ceremony, we had time to speak with Dr. Geoff Kurland and other Pulmonologists, of which I was very appreciative. Josh had strongly connected with Geoff during his many pre- and post-transplant appointments, and he had always treated Josh with respect and as an adult.

The memorial ceremony was held in a large, beautiful auditorium. On the central altar, there were candles symbolizing each child being memorialized. Children's names were read as a candle was lit for each, and someone played a guitar and sang. I was numb, but do recall Ken nudging me, telling me that my mom needed a tissue. Following the beautiful ceremony, each set of parents was given one of the candles from the beautifully displayed altar. I found it a nearly impossible task to walk down there. It was so terribly heartbreaking to have to extinguish that candle; it had such an incredible finality to it. I recall very little else about this compassionate and beautiful yet heartbreaking event. Just pain, pain, pain. I left, absolutely tortured and inconsolable.

CHAPTER 24

Processing the Grief

As Ken and I sat in the living room one evening, we both heard footsteps in the hallway coming from Josh's bedroom; the floor had a characteristic squeaky sound there in one spot. To make certain I wasn't imaging this, I asked Ken if he had heard that, and he replied "yes". I said, "Josh, if that's you, stick around. If it's anyone else, you can just go away!" A little humor, yes, but I know what we heard. There was also a flickering light in one of the lamps for a couple weeks, a sign that a spirit is attempting to contact us. I appreciated all his early attempts at saying, "It's OK mom, I'm here with you!"

Returning to work after only two weeks, I realize that I must have been quite intolerable. In deep despair, I felt unbelievably isolated, lost, aimless and hopeless. Any small comment irritated and annoyed me to no end. My feelings were raw, and in my black fog of intense pain I felt it would never be possible to be happy again. My head and heart were in excruciatingly dark places for months on end. It wasn't as if there were a cloud above me; it was like a storm was permanently attached to and surrounding my heart. I didn't know how to or if I could escape *it*. To be honest, for a very long time I wasn't sure whether I really wanted to escape it.

I remember feeling offended at work that an employee had mentioned that her son had an ear infection and went on about how terrible it was dealing with it. She repeatedly spoke about her son in my presence. Was she grateful she still had her child and had to confirm her feelings, ensuring it was within my earshot? My spirit was raw, I was deeply envious and yes, extremely resentful. How could anyone possibly complain about such simple events in their life, especially in my presence and particularly after what had recently transpired in my ragged life. Oh, what a wonderfully trivial thing to have to deal with; she had no idea! I would have given a million bucks to be in that place again. I have since accepted the fact that some people are inconsiderate and perhaps aggressively unkind due to their own fragile emotional state. Perhaps it was just a total lack of empathy. I forgive this woman for the thoughtless and seemingly deliberate infliction of pain, as she herself needed to be treated with understanding, deep compassion and empathy.

Sitting at my desk soon after my return to work, I recalled thinking, "What am I supposed to be doing?" I hadn't realized until then that I no longer knew who I was or what my mission in life was. Caring for a critically ill child had been my life's mission for many years. As any parent would feel I was responsible to keep my child healthy and well. I knew in my heart I had failed and was totally lost in a lonely home echoing with Josh's voice and laugh.

I was having difficulty organizing my thoughts. Later I learned this was a normal behavior pattern after such a loss. I found that I was extremely intolerant of what at the time I perceived as bad behavior, but now I recognize were normal day-to-day interactions and bickering. To hear laughter would instantly anger me, and I'd have to retreat to my office, quietly closing the door. I knew I could never laugh again. Thankfully later, much later, I learned that I was mistaken.

Shortly after returning to work, I was required to do a STAT portable chest x-ray in the ER. It was enormously distressing to walk into that department and to see that the patient was in the very same room where Josh had passed away only two weeks before. Though I had been doing this job for 27 years, I was so distressed that I could barely think how to perform this basic, routine task. The elderly gentleman in front of me was on oxygen, wearing a pulse oximeter and having a breathing treatment. These were essentially the same symptoms Josh had experienced when he was last on this very same bed. Well, what doesn't kill you...

Somehow finally completing my task, I left the room barely holding it together. In the hall I saw a friend who asked how I was doing. I really appreciated his concern but it was torture when I lied and replied "OK". I felt my heart implode when he asked how Josh was doing. That was only the first of several explanations of this sort that I would have to offer over the next months.

As the days and weeks passed following Josh's death, I began to understand that there would be those I would encounter who were unaware of my devastating loss. I would be called upon to give an explanation of the event. I developed a brief response, e.g., "Josh passed away two weeks ago after experiencing severe respiratory difficulties."

I found myself apologizing for the shock delivered with my words. In spite of anticipating this challenge, it in no way diminished the pain suffered when I again had to put into words the tragedy that had occurred. Naturally inquirers felt terrible that they hadn't known, and I knew in my heart that they had no intention of hurting me.

This happened multiple times at work. Each time I would go quietly into my office, close the door and totally lose it. I cried, quietly pounded my desk and asked God a lot of questions. Why couldn't it have been me?! For months, I was engulfed in a deep, dark place, unable to see my way out and was certain that truly there were no tomorrows for me. Rather, I *wanted* no tomorrows. I thought to myself' "But wait, *first* I need to buy a plot in the cemetery. Oh yes, and a coffin and a burial vault, and…oh my God, I need to talk to someone".

It first hit me as I was walking down the hall at the hospital. I came to an abrupt halt right in the middle of the corridor and experienced unexpected relief when I thought to myself, "I wouldn't care if I died right now!" I was instantly surprised at this revelation and realized that I really was quite comfortable and actually calmed by this concept. This shocking realization took place after yet again another encounter in the hallway with someone on the medical team who had attempted to resuscitate Josh in the ER.

Yes, I had anger, lots and lots of anger about all the unfinished business. This is not fair! He still had his braces on; this one disturbed me a lot. I asked him, "Now who will set our clocks and watches?" There were things to be done, life to be lived. What was God thinking? Josh was getting ready to drive and was admiring a used truck from afar. He had received his new lungs which had brought him to this point until a whole other problem knocked him off his pegs. What? I don't understand! As the anger was overwhelming me, it fed on my pain and loss and I nearly allowed it - yes, consciously - to conquer me.

It was easy to lose all optimism but there was a decision to be made. I could stay stuck in this profound grief; I could give up and "leave" or I could honor Josh's life and create an entirely new normal for myself. I would have to figure it out. Eventually I recognized that I would need to reinvent myself if I was to go on, but this took time, such a great deal of time.

In early 2017, Shawn, a schoolmate and friend of Josh spoke to me, recalling a heart-warming anecdote. When they were in the fourth grade, four or five of "the guys" had planned a sleep-over. Jan had cautioned, "Don't let him do this, be careful about that, watch out for this, make sure he does that…", etc. A few minutes later when he was alone with his friends, Josh brushed off the warnings, in essence saying something like, "Ahh, don't listen to him."

The boys had a great time camping out in the woods in a tent that night, Shawn's dad riding his four-wheeler up over the hill every couple of hours to check on them. I thanked Shawn for helping to provide Josh with an ordinary, fun-filled night of "normalcy" in his life.

Shawn also shared with me that in high school, his group of friends accompanied Josh to their classes, having threatened harm to the bully who was harassing him. When he was not feeling well, they carried his books for him. There was even a teacher who offered his classroom to the group when Josh was feeling short of breath and needed a rest.

Josh was admired and respected by his friends for living every day with integrity and intention, pushing aside the disease and his discomfort, the pain and the fear. Shawn spoke with pride, relating that Josh had signed his yearbook several years in a row, writing not just a sentence, but a paragraph that sounded as if it came from an adult.

I suspect there are many more such every-day stories, spent with good friends, that Josh never shared with me but meant so much to him.

CHAPTER 25

Difficulty Letting Go

In early March of 1997, my friend Stacy and I had thought it would be fun to go to Lily Dale, New York to get a medium's reading, so she made appointments for us. Lily Dale is described as a Center for the Science, Philosophy and Religion of Spiritualism. Many friends and acquaintances had visited the village. Walking through Lily Dale, I always sense a feeling of peace that seems to permeate the entire village; the breeze blows gently through the tall old trees, softly rustling the leaves. Ducks and geese float on the lake, people in eclectic garb stroll leisurely around the grounds, deep in quiet discussion. Others gather in rockers on porches, carrying on fascinating and mysterious conversations. It makes me want to eavesdrop and learn more!

Several weeks after Josh's passing, Stacy and I kept our appointments and trekked to Lily Dale. My unspoken yet desperate wish was that Josh would "come through". This was my first experience visiting a medium, but after hearing one of Mom's tapes, her reading sounded very specific, accurate and interesting, so our appointments had been made with the same person. I was somewhat skeptical and was cautious not to give away any clues. Well, come through he did. The medium described a young spirit around me who had recently passed. He was feeling as though a weight was on his chest and he was having difficulty breathing.

He had described Josh to a "T", right down to his chuckle, and jingling the stuff in his pockets, as he always had a tendency to do. The medium said he was with me in the car when I bumped a curb a month before and had laughed at me. Before the end of the reading, the medium asked if I'd had any recent trouble with my tires and suggested that I check them soon.

I was understandably very emotional during and after my reading and cried profusely, but it was a tremendous relief to learn that his spirit was still nearby and watching over me, confirming my feelings of him being nearby. Now, whenever I do something silly, I speak to him in my head, saying, "OK Josh, laugh it up!"

So, when our readings were complete, Stacy and I clutched our tapes and slowly walked several blocks back to the car, discussing our readings. I suppose I shouldn't have been surprised that when reaching it, we found that one tire was low, requiring prompt attention. Josh was watching out for us!

If a person can live sunk deep inside herself in a vault of darkness, pain and torment, that was surely my experience for months on end. It was as though I was inside a bottle; seeing, hearing, but unable to interact appropriately, to think about much else besides my loss. There were friends who were very supportive and had lunch with me every day for many weeks, but as time went on, this naturally and gradually slowed and then ceased. I couldn't ask them for constant attention; I couldn't let myself be so needy. Feeling utterly alone, I emotionally and physically isolated myself; the heartache and months dragged endlessly on. God Bless Ken for staying by my side as the tears, anger and tantrums continued to bubble to the surface.

Undeniably, an incredibly difficult aspect of my loss was that I had to return day after day to my place of employment where I had lost my child. There, nearly on a daily basis, passing in the hallway were the same people who were with him when he passed. Cindy, the Respiratory Therapist, a Rusty Wallace fan, for several years had teased Josh about Earnhardt and he teased her back about "Crusty" Wallace; the anesthesiologist who had been intubating him; the ER RN; they were all working to keep him alive. My gratitude for their valiant efforts will be eternal.

Three months after Josh's passing, mom was planning to take an Alaskan cruise, but would not go alone. She was 88 at the time, so that was certainly understandable. She asked me to accompany her on this wonderful trip. I really wanted nothing more than to stay home in the nest, remaining where it was safe and familiar yet sad and melancholy. But I couldn't deny her that exciting journey and reluctantly agreed. In the end, the Alaskan Inner Passage cruise was a wonderfully beautiful, distracting experience with many interesting side-trips. We both enjoyed it immensely, but on the long trip home I had time to think, feel sorry for myself and re-descend into the darkness, tears and pain.

My office, on the river side of the hospital, allowed me to hear and view every helicopter that landed on the helipad. The beat of their blades rattled the stained-glass ornaments on my window and jangled my nerves, repeatedly reminding me that there had been a chopper en route from Pittsburgh when the CPR was finally discontinued on Josh that day. I took the ornaments down, closed the blinds and didn't open them for months, an admittedly unsuccessful avoidance method for me.

Around the date of my birthday, it occurred to me one lonely night how easy it would be to close the garage door, start the car and finally be free of this unrelenting pain. It was only month 5 of a seemingly endless grieving process, but I was rational enough to recognize that first I'd need to purchase a casket, a vault, and oh yes, a plot too, right up there on the hill beside my son. I had decided I'd have to make all the pre-arrangements so I wouldn't put loved ones through what we had recently experienced. All the details would be arranged. Wouldn't "they" be pleased with me and how well organized I was? I was rationalizing my tentative, outrageous plan.

At work the next day I suddenly hit a wall. I knew Josh would be so angry if I followed through on this craziness. In the next moment, I knew I had to talk to someone about this bleak, black, deep-in-a-hole, can't-get-out sensation. I suddenly recognized that I needed to talk to a professional. I made some calls while I was feeling strong and scheduled an appointment, starting me on a lengthy grueling journey out of what I feared very easily could have been the Land of No Return. As chance would have it (or perhaps by Spirit's design), my therapist happened to be an empathetic female psychologist who had also lost her son. It was the first time I recall thinking, *"OK, maybe I'm really not the only person feeling this way."* And so began the difficult journey out of the thick, murky darkness.

I recognize that anniversaries are endless reminders for a bereaved person, not to mention a parent. The fall of 1997 was a literal firestorm of anniversaries for me, which had literally very nearly killed me. My own birthday is in October, next month would be Thanksgiving, then days later Josh's birthday, then Christmas, New Years, and on and on and on, a perpetual revolving calendar of remembrance dates. In the year 2000, Josh's death day fell on Mother's Day. Inevitable.

On Thanksgiving 2002, in a twist that was bizarre even for me, I baked a birthday cake for what would have been Josh's 21st birthday. No one could make this up, these heartbreaking Calendar Coincidences. We deal with them as best we can and that year it was Josh's birthday cake that helped me through the day. My precious niece, Sarah, helped to frost the cake. I know he was there just grinning and shaking his head.

I attended a few meetings of a local bereavement group, Welcoming Arms, for parents who had lost a child. Initially it had taken me four or five months to find the courage to go to my first meeting. My apprehension was well-founded as, when I attended the first meeting, I found I had to put into words *why* I was there, a most difficult thing at the time. At least at work I was surrounded by those who knew why I was fraying at the seams; my co-workers were loving, understanding and supportive but even then, I know for months on end I wore their patience thin.

One mother at the meeting said that it had been two years since her child's death. She was doing well. At the time, it was physically painful to hear how casual the comment sounded; I could not even imagine being in that space or how I could ever emerge from under this heavy blanket of torment and pain that relentlessly filled up my heart and very soul.

I told one sad mother who had given birth to a stillborn baby only weeks before that I felt so badly for her because she had not had the time to come to know her precious son. She replied that she felt I had suffered the greater loss, because I had known and loved my child for so long and knew him so well. I was taken aback by that comment as she was naturally approaching it from a completely different perspective. I had never thought about a child's death from this viewpoint. Both of us were mothers who had experienced the worst loss, yet each empathized with and felt the deep sorrow of the other. I didn't believe it could be possible but I felt even more depressed following each meeting. After only a few months it became too difficult to continue explaining to new members why I was in this group. Ken asked me why I continued to attend these meetings as I felt even worse when I came home. Sadly this wasn't my preferred forum for healing. For my own well-being I was compelled to drop out.

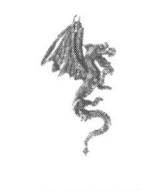

CHAPTER 26

Slogging Through the Darkness, Searching for Any Fragment of Light

One day, sitting at my desk at work in the cold winter of 1998, confused and frightened to the soul, I recognized that it was time to reinvent myself. The questions were *how, what, where?* It took two long years to formulate the answer to that. Chunks of that answer seemed to gradually fall into place here and there along the lengthy journey back to my "new" self.

The Ode to Josh blossomed into existence in March 1998. Apparently, therapy of my own making, I have written poetry and letters to Josh and my favorite, the "Ode", may be seen in a later chapter. One dark night I could hear rhyming verses in my head which literally woke me up out of a sound sleep. I felt compelled to go to the computer and get it down on "paper". I feared that I would forget the words and consequently lose a priceless gift, one I now believe had sent to me by Spirit. Why else would this message come to me in my sleep? I had never written poetry before, but for the next months, my aching soul spilled out onto paper into a lengthy, cathartic poem. I worked on it for almost six months. The ode was the beginning of my return to any semblance of normality.

April brought some distraction as I attended a mastectomy bra and breast prosthesis fitting class in Columbus, Ohio. I believe my friend Bea suggested it, in part, attempting to distract me. She must have convinced Jim, my supervisor, that I should be the person to initiate this new service in the community. In fact, it soon became a popular service with the mastectomy patients in our area. I will never forget my trip back home from Ohio. I felt Josh so strongly in the car with me and sobbed most of the agonizing five-hour drive home.

As part of my grief therapy and on a rocky road to my 'new' self, I started a local transplant support group. This endeavor was due to the continual support of Bea, who became my greatest catalyst. The motivation for this group would be to establish a connection for those in the area experiencing any transplant-related issues. I would eventually decide to name this group "Close to the Heart", as the cause as well as its reason for being would always be close to my heart.

We were very successful, having helped people of all ages in our community connect with others with similar experiences. This constructive involvement helped me enormously, and although I had lost my only child, I could funnel my grief and lessons learned into creating an organization which would positively impact others.

Close to the Heart provided support not only to those who have had a transplant and their families, but also donor families, those on a waiting list, those who may someday be a transplant candidate, and those who have lost loved ones after transplant. We helped to educate the community regarding the importance of organ donation. Emotional support of our members and community education were the two points of our Mission Statement.

Following a Close to the Heart community education engagement for the local Lion's Club about transplant and the importance of organ and tissue donation, I spoke with several of Josh's male teachers, some of them approaching me in tears, fondly remembering this special child. It was heart-warming to hear how such a young person had so profoundly impacted these adults' lives. Comments were along the lines of, "He never complained about his illness and disease". "I've never met anyone so mature and with such a positive outlook on life, despite a critical physical problem." "I have so much respect for him." "He was so pleasant to be around." "He went on despite his discomfort."

There were also similar comments from hospital staff who had either treated him or worked with him as he volunteered in the hospital snack bar. "Very courteous and well-mannered." "Always cheerful and smiling." "A wonderful person to know, a pleasure to work with." "Strong, yet kind and considerate." Josh was always small in stature but forever huge in heart.

These people may never know how comforting and affirming their words were for me.

Bea was such a wonderful friend and tremendous source of support for me. She lived literally at the edge of the cemetery where Josh's body rested. Bea was aware that my aching heart brought me to his grave daily for months on end, as my car passed by her house day after day. She reminded me that his spirit was right here at home with me and that I really didn't have to go anywhere else to gain comfort. His grave contained his body but our home contained his spirit. As winter progressed, she sensed my concern for the cold, deep snow covering over his grave. She asked me to think of it as a thick, soft white blanket, warm and insulating him from the cold. She was such a loving, compassionate and patient friend. I fondly think of her with great love and gratitude and have come to recognize and appreciate her understanding and kindness toward those she knew.

CHAPTER 27

A Child in Spirit ~

-Learning to Deal with the Death of a Child in My Own Way

Josh and his dad had mutual interests in hunting, fishing, trapping, motorcycles, snowmobiles, four-wheelers and trucks. At 15, just months before he was old enough to drive, he had already picked out the used truck he wanted to buy as soon as he had earned enough money. Over the ensuing challenging months, it was difficult for me to pass that car lot and see the vehicle he'd so longingly pointed out to me. Soon I stopped looking. Sometimes on the short drive home from work I would think, "Oh, Josh will be home, I'd better hurry." Then my heart would sink. Occasionally on the way home, I would pass his school bus coming my way and the sympathetic bus driver would wave to me. I know he was being sympathetic. It tore my heart apart seeing his bus.

I used to sit down and play songs on my guitar that Josh and I loved to sing together. How I wish I had known that the whole time Josh was here in spirit singing along with me. I would have continued to sing through my pain, and I wouldn't have quit playing and given my guitar away. Hearing his favorite songs played on the radio continue to pull at my heartstrings. Thankfully, however, they no longer provoke so much of the agony that they had for the first few years following his passing.

Josh would have graduated from high school in June of 2000. I received a special graduation invitation from the Class of 2000 and was given a yearbook that was dedicated to him. There was an empty chair up front, reserved just for him. During the ceremony, the class also recognized Close to the Heart, the transplant support group I had created in his memory. In the middle of the ceremony, dear Randy Rossman saw my distress and came to sit with me for the remainder of the time. Ann and Randy's daughter, Emily, also graduated that year. What a wonderful yet painful and challenging evening that was. I had been invited to the Rossman's after the graduation ceremony, a bittersweet occasion punctuated with wonderful memories of Josh.

The bigger, darker issues took a great deal more time. In wistful reflection, today I can think of Josh in a positive light, remembering our good times, recalling all the kudos brought to me in the years following his death by the many people who knew and respected him. I have gone beyond the days when the deeply sad and dark memories of his last day erupt like an angry, explosive volcano in my mind without warning. There were fierce dragons of my own in that darkness, etched forever in my memory as if in granite. In my heart, I sensed that if I just endured that murky time, the next day would bring a brighter outlook. Meditation and optimism thoughts seem to be weighing on the positive side of the scale so much more these days. So, in a less aggressive manner, I continue to tame my own dragons for the sake of my inner harmony and balance. I think I may have finally won the battle.

My intent here is not to impose my viewpoints and beliefs on anyone, and I certainly do not wish to offend. Everyone has their own means of rediscovering level ground after a traumatic incident. I only offer clarification of the lengthy and deeply personal and distressing process I slogged through while attempting to deal with an unimaginable event, the death of a child.

The first and second year for me was experienced as if in a thick, choking, noxious fog. Aware of the unrelenting pain I continued to deal with, about a year after Josh's passing, my brother Doug had recommended a book, *Conversations with God*, by Neale Donald Walsch. He had hoped it would provide some comfort and perhaps inspiration that I would find reassuring.

During a later telephone conversation, I joked with Doug about the reincarnation concept and stated that, "Mom better watch out, I might be the mom next time." We both laughed. I paused, reflecting on that for a few seconds and said, "Geez, maybe I was the mom *last* time!" We both burst out laughing at the irony of that statement.

That book began my journey into understanding our spiritual connections, as well as the agreements and contracts with our Soul Group (Family Group) made together before we come back into the physical world.

This clarified much for me regarding the afterlife as well as reincarnation. It also provided a great deal of comfort and led me to many other similar books. I eventually found solace in the concepts of Spiritualism and continue to study it. Some regard it as an uncomfortable subject, but for me, it is so very comforting to believe that Josh's spirit lives on and can help guide me with my life lessons if I choose to listen to his soft whispers in my ear.

Early on I read some of Sylvia Browne's books, and found comfort in the concepts she introduced. She described the writing of our charts and life contracts with our Soul Group after "returning home". It makes total sense to me, putting into context our purpose in returning to pay off our Karma and learning additional necessary Soul Lessons so that we may eventually have no need to return for additional lifetimes. Now I understand rather than wonder: how could we possibly learn all the necessary lessons in only one short lifetime?

I visited a cherished local medium, Holly Stimmell, who recognized the light in Josh's spirit. She was moved by the old soul and the lessons he offered during his short lifetime to those he knew and loved and even to those who knew him only slightly. He came to this life for only a short time, a soul contract we had agreed upon together before returning to this Earth plane. I used to ask myself, "What the heck was I thinking when I signed *that* contract?", eliciting a shake of the head and sad smile from me, and I sense, a characteristic and understanding chuckle from Josh.

He asked Holly to tell me I needed to write a book. I asked, "About what?" He responded, "About us!" And so, here it is, my dear Josh. I hope you are proud of the account I have related here and that your story and feelings are honestly and accurately reflected. In spite of making mistakes during this lifetime, I am trying to become a better person, more spiritual, empathetic, loving, tolerant, forgiving, supportive, and understanding of others' challenges and their chosen lessons during this lifetime. I need to remember that we all, for one reason or another, previously agreed to these Life-Lessons. I pray that we learn them all.

Thinking that I was past the worst stages of grief, putting our story down on paper (or rather, computer), demonstrated that unbearable and powerfully painful memories, believed to be resolved, were brought back to the surface by my writings. Numbness and denial were my methods of self-defense.

I hope that bereaved parents and others who read this book can get a sense of the spirit of Josh and how uplifting, ultimately, he has become and continues to be in my life. I want and need to honor this precious soul and his abbreviated stint here on Earth and hope I have shed a light on this old spirit. I trust that with his guidance I have adequately captured his integrity and enthusiasm for life despite life-long trials.

Frankie, my counselor, eighteen years after Josh's death asked what the block was that I encountered during the writing of this book. I recognized there were two blocks. I replied, "The time of transplant and the time surrounding his death." I immediately went into a description of the permanent image in my head that I had of his face, a picture of pure terror, when he asked me shortly following transplant whether he was going to die. This was a shocking and frighteningly atypical question coming from a thirteen-year-old. That question burrowed down in a corner of my heart, always present, occasionally nudging into my consciousness. I saw that same look just minutes before his death in the ER, but that time there were no words spoken. Frankie paused, then suggested that this was the time of our last goodbye, something just between the two of us. I instantly connected with the spirit of Josh, saw his face as it was on that day. I considered this unconventional viewpoint through a higher perspective and immediately knew it was true. His spirit was preparing to leave his body and that meaningful look, the last goodbye, would always be ours.

Through the difficult and painful process of writing this book, I pray that Josh's story inspires other heartbroken, bereaved parents to feel assured that your child in spirit would be proud of the better person you have become, honoring his or her memory, despite their brief yet delightful presence in your life. God Bless. May the Universe provide you with the peace and love of Spirit.

CHAPTER 28

Thank You

Tender and well-deserved thanks go to Jan Mickelson, Josh's father, who provided Josh with love and guidance while teaching him the skills of hunting, fishing, snowmobiles, motorcycles, four wheelers, lawn mowers, and finally, driving a truck. He provided multiple wonderful opportunities for Josh to expand his experiences and his view of the big world outside of his home. Jan drove during many of our trips to Buffalo and Pittsburgh, supporting his son during routine appointments as well as through the difficult and tragic times. Josh loved his dad deeply, was proud of him and grateful that he was able to see him any time he wished.

I would also like to acknowledge my brother, Doug Ritter, for shortly after Josh's death, recommending that I read *Conversations with God*, a book by Neale Donald Walsch. This resulted in my starting down the path to understanding the spiritual side of life and beyond. He intuitively knew that it was precisely what I needed at the time. This was a significant step toward discovering-or rediscovering-myself and my life's purpose. I extend a sincere and heartfelt thank you.

To our amazing friend, Stacy Ryan, who stuck with us through thick and thin, from the divinely wonderful, fun times through profoundly painful and unspeakably painful events, supporting and loving both Josh and me to this day: thank you and God Bless you, my forever soul-sister-friend.

Finally, to my dear husband Ken, thank you for standing by me during the deepest, darkest and most challenging and painful time of my life, for lending me strength and for allowing me to grieve in my own way and grow from the experience. I would imagine that it took an inordinate amount of patience, as I recognize that it was neither easy nor pleasant dealing with me then. I thank you more than I can say. With all of my heart and forever, I love you.

Although it just never seems sufficient, I would here like to express a deep admiration, appreciation and extend an enormous thanks to Josh's donor family. The only things we were told about Josh's donor was that she was a six-year-old little girl from the Washington DC area who had been hit by a car while riding her bicycle. I extend a deep heartfelt thank you to the family who with profound compassion saw past their own tragedy and heartbreak and offered an opportunity to help others by giving the Gift of Life. If by some extraordinary chance they happen to read these words, I wish to thank them with all my heart and soul for the ultimate gift made to Josh. I hope that somehow in their hearts they recognize our gratitude for their spirit of generosity and for giving us two more, high-quality years with our cherished son.

While it may start at a later time, soon after transplant may be the stage when many recipients and even family members themselves begin to experience feelings of guilt. You are so thankful that donated organs came in time to save your loved one's life, but at the same time you know that another family has lost a precious family member. One life lost, another one - or more - saved. Yes, just try to balance concept in your mind. Yet this notion is so much more than difficult for many recipients to wrap their heads around.

Even though you know that the donor would have nevertheless passed away, the heart overpowers the head and often the perception is reversed and some feel that, "She had to die so I could live." The bottom line is that organ donation is the ultimate gift, unquestionably the Gift of Life. How is it possible to tell a donor family the depth of gratitude for their gift, but at the same time help them understand the pain I share with them for their loss? It certainly can be a Catch 22. The key is simply to try. When you are able, write a letter and do your best to explain what that precious gift meant to your or your loved one's life.

In an attempt to increase potential organ and tissue donors and while providing community education specific to this, I have heard almost all conceivable justifications not to donate. When I ponder all those, I believe the single most memorable question posed to me has been, "What if I need them?" Taking time to consider that concept, I now respond, "God will give you new ones when you come back!"

CHAPTER 29

Love Echoes

Today I think if I could have done anything differently pre-transplant, I wish I could have prepared Josh better for what was to come. Yes, we are trading one problem for many others. The downside? Medications, lots of them, and their side effects. Susceptibility to infections, illness, rejection, setbacks, frequent hospital admissions and on and on and on…The upside? Time. Extra time. Time for life, laughter and love.

I found that friends and family avoided speaking about the death of your child, or simply asking how you are doing because they believe there's nothing left to say. Or they just avoid you because they don't know *what* to say. Is there really a right thing to say? After a week, a month, a year, what can anyone say? What comfort can be offered? I believe their fear is about hurting you, reminding you of the pain. I'll say this now, that no, there is no greater pain than losing a child, but you can't *remind* me of it. It's never gone, it's always there. It is in the forefront of my mind. Just to know you are thinking of me is enough, for which I am grateful. Your beautiful shared happy memories are delightful. "I am thinking of you" is more than sufficient for a grieving parent to hear. Make no mistake: I am so very grateful to have had the experience of Josh for the years that I did. I would not have missed that rewarding experience for all the money in the world. Literally.

And finally, I dealt with my pain by changing *me*. Realizing that my life's mission had completely changed in the space of one fleeting hour, for months I struggled to find my reason for being, for *staying*. Why am I here? Resisting the temptation to give in to increasing depression and desperation was a massive challenge. Just barely seeing through the fog in my mind, I realized that my goals, my purpose for being if I were to stay, would have to be rewritten and I was the only one to do it.

A parent cannot endure this experience and expect to be forever unchanged. The personal decision to be made is exactly what those changes will be and how the many challenges will be met.

CHAPTER 30

"Ode to Josh"

Written March – August, 1998
-Debbie Sumner, Mom

It's been almost a year, I've been thinking of you,
It hurts as much now as when my loss was new.
I remember that day, the terror, the pain,
The weight on my chest, in that ER again.

When they felt for a pulse but could not find one,
They made me leave that room; then I knew I was done.
My heart, how it pounded; I screamed in my head,
"I can't lose this boy, who'll care for me?" I said.

"IT DOESN'T LOOK GOOD"… chilling words that will forever
Sound in my mind, allow my poor heart to never
Forget the worst thing ever said to a mom or a dad;
I can't imagine anything else ever being so sad.

"Sensei Rick" was there too, trying, despite his own grief
To console us, our loss, so enormously deep.
A loss, I've learned, from talking with so many
Is shared by all who knew you, even just barely.

I felt the wrench in my gut, the spin in my head,
The grip on my heart, and wished I were dead.
I knew for weeks after, this was only a dream,
Surely, I'd wake up soon; all was not what it seemed.

Driving home in shock, I was so very amazed
How everyone else acted absolutely unfazed.
Didn't they know my whole world just fell apart?
Heaven's reclaimed angel went home to create a new chart.

That morning I returned home in utter disbelief
My heart feeling black, sunk so deep in its grief,
A FedEx box at the door delivered your new beeper
For your next set of lungs, borrowed from their last keeper.

I talked to Geoff on the phone; he was to see you in the 'Burgh that day.
He wondered what had happened, in my shock, I couldn't say.
From the hospital, in pain, we'd just returned,
Our friends down in Pittsburgh had all just now learned

Of your fate - today you would not be down,
We'd soon have to lay our dear son in the ground.
How could this happen? It's just not right
That our sweet child is gone; so empty, so dark, so hollow the night.

So many who loved you - Gram, Stace, Candy and Dad…
So many in shock, thinking of fun we'd all had.
Suddenly all over, now how could this be?
I should be up there with you, or you down here with me!

I remember the big bear that you'd shot, standing tall, dark and scary
And how the taxidermist took too long to get it ready.
Your braces, still on, still doing their work, though not yet done
How could God call you now, so much left to do - work, play and fun?

The truck you promised to work so hard for,
To drive in only six months, well, that's out the door!
It sat there on the lot, still at the dealer,
Waiting for you to climb in and drive; your very own four-wheeler.

You went to Charlotte with Make-A-Wish and Dad,
Met Earnhardt and others, a huge dream that you'd had.
You saw racecars, met drivers and owners, had your picture taken.
They autographed your jacket and hat; you were honored yet shaken.

My little black belt, I bragged far and wide,
Began young winning trophies, I boasted with pride.
Teaching others your skills in and out of the dojo
Everyone who met you loved and respected you so.

Craig, your "big brother", hurt so much from this…
Remembers the fun things you both did, the guns and their clips.
The cardinal incident - oh, you learned much that day
From this big guy you admired, "Please, Mom, can't we stay?"

You cried when we left him; you both wrote back and forth,
You looked forward to next time, not knowing you both
Would never set eyes on each other again,
No more laughter or shared secrets - too soon, a fallen friend.

He carried you high on those strong shoulders so wide,
You were proud and cocky up there, on your tall ride.
Lifted up like a feather, not a care did you have,
In heaven already, with him you were even more brave.

You wanted to be just like Craig; big strong and wise,
But you were so darn small and thin; a giant in disguise.
You didn't know the strength and the courage you had,
He admires your determination and misses you; he's so very sad.

He's sad that you're gone from us, taken all too soon,
He'll miss all the things that you both liked to do.
I hope precious memories of you get him through
As they help all those many who admire and still love you.

You'd been put back on the waiting list, much to your dismay
And came home disappointed, sad, that last-appointment day.
So, we decided to take the Blazer and drive over "The Falls."
We laughed out loud (crying inside); our spirits had hit a solid rock wall.

You still clearly remembered the pain, the hospital bed,
Your intense fear that you'd soon be dead.
I still see the look of terror on your face soon after transplant,
The very same one I saw that last day, as if to say, "Mom, I can't…"

Later, Cindy shared with me what you'd said when I left that room
To reach out for help in Pittsburgh, those rip-your-heart-out words of gloom:
"Don't tell my mom, I don't want her to cry".
Your concern was for me, though you knew to heaven you'd soon fly.

I thought I'd had a pact with God; He went back on his word.
If he'd give you your health (what a double-edged sword),
I'd trade places in a heartbeat, give you all the wealth;
The jewels of no worries; the gift of your breath.

The gems of no pills, no pain, tubes or knife,
No watching your struggle for breath, I'd give you my life!
Can't I trade with him, O God, please just this one,
My life on this earth for that of my son?

What good was I, unable to keep you alive?
Wasn't that my job, to protect and provide?
God, I so need that wonderful, great child
To be back in my house, in my arms, by my side.

I wanted so badly once more to hold you,
To talk, and to comfort and be fearless too,
Or at least say goodbye one very last time;
Never given the chance, my grief is honed fine.

I needed so much to hear your sweet voice, then…
Dreamed I heard you say "Mom", then "MOM!" once again.
You stood there so close, right by my bed,
Scared me nearly to death 'til your familiar chuckle echoed 'round in my head.

In your short lifetime you offered so much, so true,
So much more to me than I could ever give you.
Perfect gift from God but not so well heeded,
Surprise child I didn't realize I wanted, but profoundly needed.

You taught me no longer to be selfish or vain;
Dear, precious child, I tried to ease all your pain.
To talk, boast and brag about all you had done;
But ultimately, you and you alone were the important one.

God, please let us trade places, I've been here long enough.
Let my near-man come back; make his times here less tough.
Josh, you took my heart with you when you suddenly left,
I don't know how to survive, absolutely bereft.

But I know if I show up in heaven too early
Before I've been able to honor your memory,
You'd surely kick butt for my giving up on life,
'Cause my job down here now is to lead, help overcome strife.

After the pain, the close calls, that awful chopper trip,
Damn treatments, cutting, staples and those surgical clips,
The meds, breathless nights, protocols closely followed,
You paid so very dearly; it leaves my heart hollowed.

We did what we should, you took all those pills!
The biopsies, tests, x-rays, all such steep hills.
You endured all their probing, my pushing, their rules,
None of this was enough, God, you would not be fooled.

So many weeks in hospitals, together we spent.
Guess that wasn't enough…oh, please let me vent
My deep pain, my frustration, with all this I thought
A good life several times over that surely, you'd bought.

So many reminders roam around work; there they stay.
Doctors, nurses and techs tried to save you that day.
Now the choppers fly in, send my window a-rattle,
They remind me of you as you fought your final battle.

To the hospital the last chopper from Pittsburgh fast flew,
But not fast enough, my pain grew and grew.
You lay there, finally resting, no more pain and at peace,
We stood there beside you, questioning how your life could have ceased.

You'd accepted her gift of lungs to extend your best times,
And after you'd done your finest, made an offering in kind.
You gave up your eyes so a baby boy who coos
Could see his whole life through your own baby-blues.

Memories of that day never stop - it's unending doom.
Words that were spoken, friends' faces, profound gloom!
Sometimes I still don't believe that this happened, just a dream, I am sure.
I'll wake up any time; now you'll be here - my sweet cure.

The chest film I did, only two weeks later *was in that same room.*
Poor old man, short of breath, all tubed up, made my head boom,
It tore my heart out – I nearly lost my cool head,
I could only think of you going to heaven from that very same bed.

Leaving there, next door, I saw a friend who had cared,
He asked how you were; that day my heart was not to be spared.
I told him what happened, our loss was so great.
He felt bad for asking. How much longer do I carry this weight?

The week after you left, Make-A-Wish called about a new NASCAR thing.
They knew that you'd love it, so they gave us a ring.
They had yet not heard about our terrible loss;
They thought of this gift only for my beloved Josh.

The magazines of motocross, of transplants, of guns
Continued to come, so I called them one by one.
I asked please, quit sending a monthly reminder.
You were no longer here to read them; I could phrase it no kinder.

Then came a friend from out of town who hadn't heard,
She asked how I was, and about you too, how you fared.
My pain was so great, but that, I knew I must weather.
Escaping back to my office, I tried to put my shattered heart back together.

I know you would like my new best-friend man,
He's even sometimes a Dale Earnhardt fan!
Though you met just a few times, he's your kind of guy
Honest, forthright and kind…and a little bit shy.

Now please Josh, lend your strength, your sharp wit;
Your courage, your humor, your immense spirit;
The jokes and the laughs, that twinkle in your eye,
The love of your friends, (now I'll make *me* cry!).

Give me the strength that helped you through pain, fear and dread.
Help me help those, who in our shoes must now tread
Through the months of their sickness, remind me of you,
All the worries, the terror, torment you went through.

Can I bear my own pain, be strong for them all?
I'm not sure I have it, Josh: Oh, please give me a call!
For those who need lungs, a kidney, heart, liver...
Can I do this for them? Memories make me quiver.

Help me be strong, keep your love in my head.
Some of these new friends hang on just by a thread.
Give me the strength which kept you alive
For so long; the doctors were amazed you'd survived.

Give to me, my young Sensei, sweet son almost driving,
That which sustained you, kept you constantly striving
For life, fun and laughter; hunting, fishing, four-wheelers,
Motorcycles and friends, those crazy snowmobilers.

Look down on me from your special place up there in heaven,
Lend me your clarity, your now crystal-clear vision.
Gaze down upon me, lend me your strength;
You will see that I give it my all, going to any length.

Just to know that you're up there in heaven looking out,
Those eyes watching and guiding me, stumbling blindly about,
Forgiving life's errors, flaws and faults in each,
Helps my heart find a comforting corner of peace.

For all those deer, the squirrels, bear, and turkey,
For that man, we knew in our hearts was so "jerky".
Give me your strength, your humor, and power of life,
After this, I will never know comparable strife.

To Alaska with Dad, for hunting with bow,
Hopes and plans that you made; yeah honey, I know.
For all those things you so badly needed to do,
You ran out of time, so now I offer this humble tribute to you:

Greatest person I've known, the best kid that I've met,
The closest to God on this Earth I'll ever get!
So honored to have known you, only child of mine,
Wish it could've been me; let you stay here, feeling fine.

Up there greeting children leaving Earth at too young an age,
Helping them adjust to their new life, to turn their own page.
Teach them as you did me, to love without doubt,
Show them white beaming light, your joyful, "visual shout".

If all our precious memories make a kings' palace bright,
In heaven, there's a throne (or at least a motorcycle) in dazzling white light.
If all these things exist, as I know they must, then you surely fit,
And there's a place near the Pearly Gates, on your bike, where you sit.

With unending Love and Respect,
Mom

CHAPTER 31

"Why Does It Happen?"

Written May 1997 by a friend, Amanda Meneo,
sister of Eric, who was a close friend of Josh's

Why does it happen
out of the blue?

Why does it happen
to me and to you?

I knew it would happen,
but I hoped not to I,
because people like us,
aren't supposed to die.

All death adds is pain & sorrow,
that won't go away
by the day after tomorrow.

It devastates family & friends
and punctures the heart
where the hurt never ends.

Why does it happen
out of the blue?

Why does it happen
to me and you?

~In loving memory of Josh Mickelson, who passed away on May 14th, 1997.

CHAPTER 32

"The Dragon Asked"
-Donna Mutzabaugh

The dragon asked:

Won't you come to my domain where we will play and just have fun?

We'll throw a ball and bat it, and romp and jump and run.

We'll race across the plains; you astride with boots and hat.

There may be many good things but not as good as that.

We will live with creatures wild; raccoons and bear and deer.

We'll explore the forest dark, adventurers without fear.

We will wade in a stream; trickling water through our toes.

Forgetting and not caring 'bout time and how it goes.

Then at night we will lie watching sky and stars

And hope of going into space to Jupiter and Mars.

We won't have a bedtime and problems will not borrow

Happy dreams await us and great plans for tomorrow.

Without hesitation the boy said "Yes";

And the dragon smiled his dragon smile, turned and led the way.

APPENDIX A

Organs for Transplant

The Center for Organ Recovery &Education (CORE), based in Pittsburgh, Pennsylvania, is a regional organ procurement organization (OPO). It is important to note that one organ, tissue and cornea donor can save or enhance the lives of up to 75 recipients. The following information is taken from CORE's website, www.core.org.

Liver
- The liver is the largest organ in the body, responsible for crucial functions such as the breakdown of harmful substances in our blood and the production of bile that aids in digestion. It allows the body to filter medications and toxins, and metabolize carbohydrates, fats and proteins.
- Liver failure can be caused by viral infections, genetic disorders or alcoholism. These liver diseases lead to cirrhosis, which creates scar tissue that blocks the flow of blood and impedes its functions.
- Liver transplants are the only hope for long-term survival for patients with end-stage liver disease.
- Most liver transplants involve transplanting the entire liver. In this case, the diseased liver is removed and replaced with a healthy one. However, it is possible to transplant part of a liver, as the organ can regenerate itself within the body. This is how it is possible for people to be living liver donors, as both the transplanted lobe and the donor's lobe will grow in their respective bodies.
- A liver from an adult donor can often be split and transplanted into two people.

Heart
- The heart is the body's hardest-working muscle. It is located behind the breastbone, between the lungs, and pumps blood throughout the body. Deoxygenated blood flows from the heart to the lungs, where it gives up waste and is freshly oxygenated. From there, the blood returns to the heart and is pumped to the rest of the body. Like any muscle, the heart can be subject to fatigue, especially if it has been weakened by a number of cardiovascular diseases. If the heart experiences enough damage, patients may need a heart transplant. A heart transplant is usually needed following medical conditions such as coronary artery disease, cardiomyopathy or weakening of the heart muscle.
- Today, heart transplants and combination heart/lung transplants are almost routine operations. These transplants have saved thousands of lives.
- For patients who await a heart transplant, donation is the key to saving their life as the severity of the weakened heart is critical. If a heart transplant is not immediately available, the only option for the patient is to be assisted with a mechanical heart called an LVAD (left ventricular assist device), which can be surgically implanted to maintain blood pumping until a transplant is available.

Kidney
- The primary function of the kidneys is to remove waste from the body through the production of urine. The kidneys also help regulate blood pressure, blood volume and the chemical (electrolyte) composition of the blood. Patients who need kidney transplants have suffered from some form of kidney failure, which can be a result of diabetes, high blood pressure or a number of diseases that can be inherited. If left untreated, kidney failure can be fatal.
- On average, patients on the transplant waiting list wait five years for a kidney transplant.
- Kidney transplants are the most frequently performed and the most successful organ transplant procedures.
- While most people are born with two kidneys, we can survive with only one. That is why individuals are able to be living kidney donors and help save the life of a loved one or stranger.

Intestine
- Intestines are often transplanted into children and young adults with severe digestive disorders. In children, the small intestine is often transplanted in combination with the liver, stomach and pancreas — a multi-visceral transplant.
- Both the small and large intestines are part of the digestive system. They help the body to absorb nutrients, and they are also charged with removing waste products. Together, they run about 25 feet long. The intestines are separated into the upper part (the small intestine) and the lower part (the large intestine). The small intestine aids in digestion and extracts nutrients from the food we eat. The large intestine is wider than the small intestine and handles absorption of water so that it can be placed into the blood stream. While the large intestine is not absolutely necessary to sustain life, problems with the small intestine can present the need for a transplant. Conditions that create problems for the small intestine include short bowel syndrome caused by conditions like tumors, Crohn's disease and other inflammatory bowel diseases, or congenital heart defects.

Lung
- Lung transplants give renewed life to pulmonary hypertension patients and young people afflicted with cystic fibrosis.
- Our lungs are responsible for absorbing oxygen into the bloodstream and removing carbon dioxide from the body. The lungs are comprised of five lobes — three on the right and two on the left. A person is able to live with only 30% lung capacity, but people who have sustained even more damage require a transplant. Reasons for lung damage include hereditary issues, smoking or environmental pollution.
- Timely transplants are crucial for potential lung transplant recipients, who often require round-the-clock oxygen while on the waiting list. With lung transplants, living donors are possible. Two donors can each offer a lobe of their own, and both lobes are transplanted into the patient.

Pancreas
- Individuals who have severe complications from diabetes can benefit from pancreas or combined kidney/pancreas transplants. Pancreas transplants offer hope to patients with type 1 diabetes.
- As part of the digestive system, the pancreas produces insulin, a hormone that transforms sugar into fuel for the body. It also produces enzymes that break down fat, protein and carbohydrates during digestion. A person with a poorly functioning pancreas has a surplus of sugar in the blood because the body is not producing enough insulin. Excess sugar in the blood can lead to kidney failure, heart disease, stroke or even death. Many people with pancreas failure also have renal failure. The most common cause of pancreas disease is type 1 diabetes, previously referred to as juvenile diabetes. An experimental treatment of this disease involves transplantation of islet cells. These insulin-producing islet cells are isolated from the donor's pancreas and injected into the patient's liver, where they begin to produce insulin for the recipient. In the United States, doctors frequently transplant a kidney with the pancreas.

APPENDIX B

Tissues for Transplant

Much like organ donation, tissue donation can dramatically change someone's quality of life or even save someone's life. A person has the ability to donate a variety of tissues.

Corneas
Donated corneas help to restore sight to those who are blind or who have suffered eye trauma of some sort.

Bone/Tendon
Bone and tendon transplants can help someone avoid amputation if their bones or tendons have been adversely affected by tumors, trauma or infection.

Heart Valves
A donated heart valve can restore heart function. Heart valves transplanted into a young patient's body will grow with that person, enabling him or her to avoid additional surgeries.

Vein/Artery
Doctors can transplant veins and arteries into a transplant recipient's body during coronary artery bypass surgery. For those suffering with diabetes, a transplanted vein or artery can restore blood flow to a limb that was not receiving enough blood, thereby avoiding the need for amputation.

Skin

People who have suffered burns or trauma can greatly benefit from skin transplants because the newly donated skin can protect the body from infection and promote healing. Doctors can also use donated skin to repair cleft palates or for mastectomy reconstruction.

Marrow

A healthy blood system is always making new blood-forming cells. These are necessary for survival. If the body begins making diseased cells or not enough healthy cells, a bone marrow or cord blood transplant may be the best treatment and only potential cure. A bone marrow transplant can save the life of someone battling leukemia, lymphoma or another blood cancer.

APPENDIX C

Donation Myths

According to CORE, the following are common myths regarding organ and tissue donation:

MYTH: If I am in an accident and medical personnel know that I'm a registered donor, they won't try to save my life.
TRUTH: The number one priority is to save every life. Paramedics, nurses and doctors will do **everything** possible to save your life. CORE is only notified after all life-saving efforts have failed.

MYTH: There is no difference between being brain dead and being in a coma.
TRUTH: Brain death is the medical, legal and moral determination of death. To verify brain death, a series of tests are performed over a period of time and more than one diagnosis is required before the patient's family is presented with the opportunity to donate. There is no recovery from brain death.

MYTH: My religion does not support donation.
TRUTH: All major religions consider donation to be an individual decision or support it as the final act of love and generosity toward others.

MYTH: The rich and famous receive preferential treatment on the transplant waiting list.
TRUTH: Financial and celebrity status do not determine who receives a transplant. A national computer network, maintained by the United Network for Organ Sharing (UNOS), matches organs according to height, weight and blood type, followed by medical urgency and then time accrued

on the waiting list. Age, race, gender, religious affiliation or financial status are not factors determining who receives a transplant.

MYTH: I am too old to register to become an organ donor.
TRUTH: There is no age limit for organ donation. Every potential donor is evaluated on a case-by-case basis at the time of their death to determine which organs and tissues are suitable for donation.

MYTH: My organs aren't of any value because of my medical illnesses.
TRUTH: Few illnesses or conditions prevent someone from being a donor. At the time of death, CORE reviews medical and social histories to determine suitability. Although someone may not be able to donate blood, it does not always prevent the individual from donating organs and tissues.

MYTH: Organs go to people who didn't take care of theirs.
TRUTH: Organs go to people who were born with or developed diseases that have caused organ failure. Less than 5% of people awaiting transplant have damaged their organ through substance abuse and they must achieve and sustain sobriety before they can be listed for transplant.

MYTH: My family will have to pay for costs related to my donation.
TRUTH: Donors and their families are not responsible for any costs related to donation. All costs are incurred by the organ procurement organization.

MYTH: Organs are bought and sold on the black market.
TRUTH: In alliance with the National Organ Transplant Act, the buying and selling of organs and tissue is illegal. Additionally, due to the complexity of organ transplantation, necessary involvement from highly trained medical professionals, the process of matching donors with recipients, the need for modern medical facilities, and the support required for transplantation, it would be impossible for organs to be bought or sold on the black market.

MYTH: The recipient will learn my identity.
TRUTH: Information about an organ donor is only released to the recipient if the family of the donor requests or agrees to it. Otherwise, a patient's privacy is maintained for both donor families and recipients.
www.core.org/understanding-donation/dispelling-the-myths/

APPENDIX D

Living Donation

Giving the gift of a kidney, a lobe of a lung, or a portion of the liver, pancreas or intestine, living donors offer patients an alternative to waiting on the national transplant list for an organ from a deceased donor. The number of living organ donors is more than 6,000 per year, and one in four of these donors are not biologically related to the recipient.

What is Living Donation?
The majority of organ donations occur after a donor has died. However, living donation is possible with certain organs and tissues, enabling doctors to save more people in desperate need of a transplant. Living kidney and liver donors can range from family members and friends to anonymous individuals if they meet the requirements to donate.

Advantages of Living Donation
When doctors are able to transplant an organ from one family member to another, the genetic match often decreases the risk of rejection.
Because it is a living donation, the procedure can be scheduled at a convenient time for both the donor and recipient.
Kidney transplant recipients often see an immediate return of normal function.
Types of Organs Supplied by Living Donors
Kidney – Individuals can donate one of their two kidneys to a recipient, making this the most common form of living organ donation. Although donors will see a decrease in kidney function after donation, their remaining kidney will function properly in working to remove waste from the body.

Liver (lobe) – People can donate one of two lobes of their liver. The liver cells in the remaining lobes of the liver regenerate after the donation until the organ has regrown to almost its original size. This occurs in both the donor and recipient

Lung (lobe) – Lung lobes do not regenerate, but individuals can donate a lobe of one lung. Living lung donation occurs when two adults give the right and left lower lobes (from each respectively) to a recipient. The donor's lungs must be the right volume and size to be a correct match.

Matching Donors and Transplant Patients

Paired donation or paired exchange involves two pairs of potential living kidney donors and transplant candidates who are not compatible. The two candidates "trade" donors so that each candidate receives a kidney from a compatible donor.

Kidney donor waiting list exchange occurs when a living donor who is incompatible with the intended transplant candidate donates to an anonymous candidate on the waitlist so the intended candidate can be given higher priority on the waitlist.

Blood type incompatible donation occurs when a transplant candidate receives a kidney from a living donor with an incompatible blood type. To decrease the risk of rejection of the donated organ, candidates receive specialized medical treatment before and after the transplant.

Positive cross-match donation involves a living donor and a transplant candidate who are incompatible because antibodies (a protein substance) in the candidate will immediately react against the donor's cells, causing loss of the transplant. Specialized medical treatment is provided to the candidate to prevent rejection.

Certain living donation options may not be available at all transplant centers. Contact transplant centers directly for information on specific programs.

History of Living Donation

The first successful living donation took place when, in 1945, Dr. Joseph Murray transplanted a healthy kidney from Ronald Herrick into his twin brother, Richard. He had been suffering from chronic kidney failure, but lived a healthy life after the transplant until his death from causes not related to the transplant. Ronald, his living donor brother, lived for 56 years after the surgery until his death in 2010.

Altruistic Kidney Donation
Living kidney donors who are not related to or known by the recipient are known as non-directed donors. This type of selfless donation can also be referred to as altruistic or anonymous non-directed kidney donation.

In this case, the transplant center determines how the donor's kidney will be used. Non-directed donors may help multiple transplants occur by donating to a paired donation program where their altruistic donation may be useful to a "chain" of donations. It is important to note that living donors are never paid – it is illegal to donate an organ for profit under the National Organ Transplant Act of 1984, and transplant centers are prohibited from accepting living donors who have been pressured to donate.

When the organ recipient knows the potential donor, the recipient's insurance pays for clinical evaluations to ensure they are in the best possible state of health to move forward with the donation. If you are an altruistic donor without a known recipient, your insurance provider will most likely refuse to pay for your evaluation tests. Luckily, most local transplant centers cover these expenses. Please visit CORE's website to view links to all kidney transplant centers within the CORE service area.

To Become a Living Donor
The health and safety of a living donor is the most important priority in any transplant procedure involving a living donor. Emotionally and physically, living donors must be in top condition.
Living Donors Must...
Donate voluntarily. At any time during the donation process a living donor may change his or her mind. This decision will be kept confidential.
Be in good health overall with normal organ function and anatomy.
Be physically fit. In most cases, donors should not have high blood pressure, diabetes, cancer, kidney disease or heart disease.
Not be paid. It is illegal to pay or be paid for a donation under the National Organ Transplant Act of 1984 and state law.
18-60 years old (in most cases).

Complete clinical evaluations beyond the initial donation criteria to confirm compatibility with a recipient. These include physical and psychological evaluations.

Give informed consent. Transplant centers must ensure that the prospective donor has been informed regarding the aspects of living donation and possible outcomes.

Types of Living Donors Directed Donation

Related Living Directed Donation: Includes healthy blood relatives of candidates:

Brothers and sisters

Parents

Children over 18 years of age

Other blood relatives (aunts, uncles, cousins, half-brothers and -sisters, nieces and nephews)

Non-related Directed Donation: These are healthy, unrelated living donors who are emotionally close to transplant candidates, including:

Spouses

Relatives through marriage

Close friends

Co-workers, neighbors or other acquaintances

Non-directed/Altruistic Donation: These living donors are not related and unknown to the recipient. Altruistic donors make their donation for purely selfless reasons and are sometimes called anonymous donors.

Paired Exchange Donation: This system enables a living donor to initiate a chain of transplants to the benefit of more than one person in need. Non-directed kidney donors who wish to donate to anyone waiting for a kidney can be included in paired exchange donation programs.

The Decision to Donate

The decision to donate is very personal, and potential donors should make their decision with all the available information to make an informed choice. Donation must be a voluntary decision that is free from pressure of any kind.

A living donor may change his or her mind at any point in the donation process. This decision and any reasons will be kept strictly confidential. Potential donors should consider the possible health effects of donation as well as the life-saving potential for the transplant recipient.

Usually, a donor's life returns to normal within four to six weeks after the surgery, but because of all the effects on donors, particularly unknown long-term effects, the federal government does not actively encourage any individual to make a living donation. They do recognize the wonderful gift provided to transplant recipients, and through the Division of Transplantation, Health Resources Services Administration and U.S. Department of Health and Human Services, the federal government works to support living donors.

Medical expenses for living donation are generally covered by the recipient's insurance plan. Transplant centers are required to charge recipients an "acquisition fee" upon receiving a transplant, which covers the donor's pre-donation clinical evaluations, the transplant procedure and postoperative care, also referred to as "donor protocol." Other costs outside of this protocol are not covered. More extensive and detailed information about the financial aspects of the procedure can be provided by the transplant center.

Who Makes a Good Donor?
Ultimately, a transplant center has the definitive say on whether or not a person can become a living donor. A person who wishes to make a living donation is carefully screened for the best possible physical and psychological outcome for both the donor and the recipient.

Resources for Living Donation
Contact the potential recipient's transplant center to receive more information or be tested as a potential living donor for someone you know. Ask to speak with the transplant coordinator who will be able to provide you with additional information and get you started in the donation process.

Visit websites below for additional information:
Kidney Paired Donation Resources:
National Living Donor Assistance Center (NLDAC)
Transplant Living
Alliance for Paired Donation (APD)
National Kidney Registry (NKR)
United Network for Organ Sharing
U.S. Federal Health Resources and Services Administration

American Society for Transplantation
National Kidney Foundation
Living Kidney Donor Network (LKDN)

https://www.core.org/understanding-donation/living-donation/

APPENDIX E

Support Organizations

- CORE (Center for Organ Recovery & Education): www.core.org
- MOTTEP (Minority Organ Tissue Transplant Education Program): www.core.org/community/community-education/multicultural/
- Link to register to be an organ donor: www.core.org/register/
- Donate Life: donatelife.net/
- Unos.org
- Organdonor.gov
- Bethematch.org

APPENDIX F

Further Reading

- Rosof, B., *The Worst Loss, How Families Heal from the Death of a Child*, Henry Hold and Company, Inc., 1994.
- Rando, T. A., *Grieving: How to Go on Living When Someone You Love Dies*, Jossey-Bass, Inc. Publishers, 1988.
- Rando, T. A., *Parental Loss of a Child*, Research Press Company, 1986.
- Anderson, G., Martin, J., Romanowski, P., Our Children Forever, PAR Bookworks, Ltd, 1994.
- Konigsberg, R. D., *The Truth About Grief: The Myth of Its Five Stages as the New Science of Loss*, Simon and Schuster Paperbacks, 2011.
- Walshttps://smile.amazon.com/Faber-Castell-Metallic-Texture-Kit-Crafting/dp/B01B5BKD0Y/ref=sr_1_31?keywords=crafting+media&qid=1567437712&s=arts-crafts&sr=1-31ch, N. D., *Conversations with God, an Uncommon Dialogue, Book 2*, Hampton Roads Publishing Company, Inc., 1997.
- Van Praagh, J., *Growing Up in Heaven, The Eternal Connection Between Parent and Child*, HarperCollins Publishers, 2011.
- Norris, D. I., *On Dragonfly Wings, A Skeptic's Journey to Mediumship*, Axis Mundi Books, 2014.
- Sylvia, Claire, with Novak, William, *A Change of Heart, a Memoir*, Little, Brown and Company.

ABOUT THE AUTHOR

Debbie Sumner, first-time author, retired from Warren General Hospital in Warren Pennsylvania after a 43-year career in Imaging Services, 33 of those as a manager. She lives in Warren with her husband Ken and their beloved adopted Black Labs, Bailey and Dakota. Josh was an only child. Ken has two adult sons.

In October of 1999, a year and a half after Josh's death, Debbie established a local transplant support group, "Close to the Heart". This group was founded to honor Josh's memory and to help local people and their families with much-needed emotional support before and after transplant.

After 20 wonderfully rewarding years, Close to the Heart Transplant Support Group was dissolved to allow others who may be interested take up the reins, supporting local people who are on the organ and tissue transplant and donation track.

Debra S. Sumner
4 Hyatt Drive
Warren, PA 16365
Home: (814) 726-1499
Email: tamingjoshsdragon@gmail.com